A GLIMPSE OF
VETERINARY EDUCATION IN INDIA
(A Service to the Profession)

A GLIMPSE OF VETERINARY EDUCATION IN INDIA

(A Service to the Profession)

By :

Prof. (Dr.) Jitendra Singh Bhatia

B.V.Sc & A.H., M.Sc. (A.I.I.M.S.) Ph.D.
Former ADG (Education, Development and Planning)
ICAR and Professor of Veterinary Physiology
Presently Professor and Head of Veterinary Physiology and Biochemistry,
Khalsa College of Veterinary and Animal Sciences
Amritsar-143 002 (Punjab)

SSPH

SATISH SERIAL PUBLISHING HOUSE

403, Express Tower, Commercial Complex, Azadpur, Delhi-110033 (India)
Phone : 011-27672852, Fax : 91-11-27672046
E-mail : info@satishserial.com, hkjain1975@yahoo.com
Website : www.satishserial.com

Published by :

SATISH SERIAL PUBLISHING HOUSE

403, Express Tower, Commercial Complex, Azadpur, Delhi-110033 (INDIA)
Phone : 011-27672852 Fax : 91-11-27672046
E-mail : info@satishserial.com, hkjain1975@yahoo.com

ISBN 978-93-85055-34-8

Typeset at: Harminder Kharb *for* Laxmi Art Creation
Printed at: Salasar Imaging Systems, Delhi-110035

Dedicated

To

My Beloved

Parents

who remained

great inspirational

forces to shape

my life

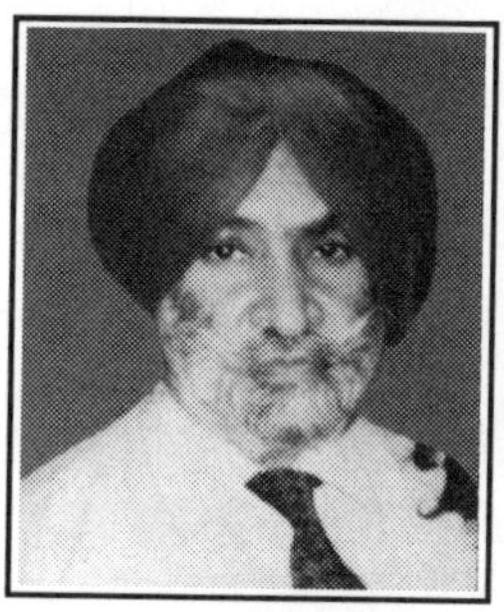

Late Sardar
Rawel Singh Bhatia

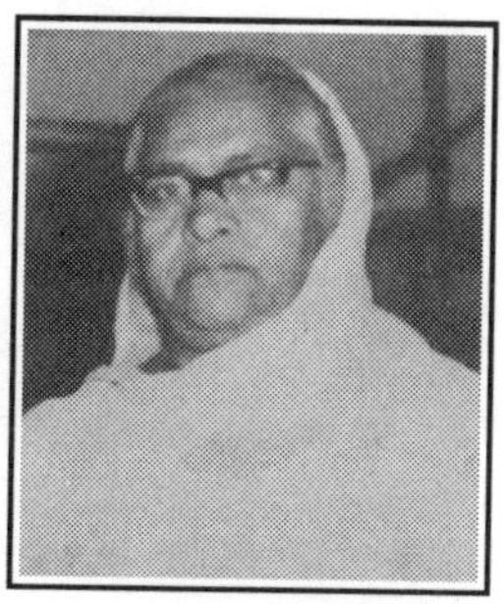

Late Sardarni
Swarn Kaur

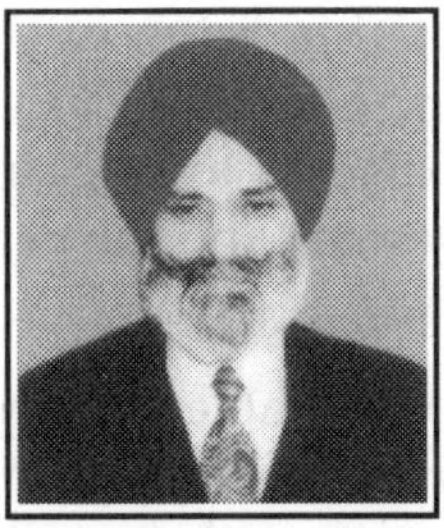

Sardar Rajender Mohan Singh Chhina
Honorary Secretary
Khalsa College Governing Council, Amritsar

FOREWORD

It is with pride I am presenting an introductory note on the book entitled "A Glimpse on Veterinary Education in India" authored by Prof. Jitendra Singh Bhatia, Professor of Veterinary Physiology and Academic Coordinator at the Khalsa College of Veterinary and Animal Sciences, Amritsar. Prof. Bhatia has made a beginning by bringing out his maiden publication from recently established veterinary college under the aegis of the Khalsa College charitable society (Estt. 1892) at Amritsar. The college will continue to strive to bring relevant publications on different aspects of livestock sector.

The author, in this book has compiled the gist of his lifelong learning and experiences acquired during the 50 years while working in different capacities as educationist, scientist and academic managers in universities, ICAR etc. He has the distinction of serving in private system of veterinary education for the last 12-years probably, one amongst a few in the country.

This book provides composite analysis on the status of veterinary education in the country. The author has tried to construct a road map starting from the development taken place right from beginning of human civilization to the progressive transformations occurred over the times. This profession has made tremendous stride by garnering supports from successive governments, untiring efforts on the part of the professionals and the participations of stake holders especially the farming community. Forward looking measures suggested by Prof. Bhatia on certain issues/ concerns would definitely make the veterinary educational system more vibrant, productive and conducive for growth.

I am confident that this book will provide building bricks for furtherance of veterinary education to enable the country to produce human resource that is expected to be equipped with the knowledge and skills for the welfare of livestock and the peasants whose sustenance source is mainly animal husbandry.

The Khalsa College charitable society greatly appreciate the efforts of Prof. Bhatia and other contributors for this novel act of bringing this book that carries information that will be useful in revamping the educational system.

I wish all the success to this venture.

Sardar Rajinder Mohan Singh Chhina
Honorary Secretary
Khalsa College Governing Council
Amritsar

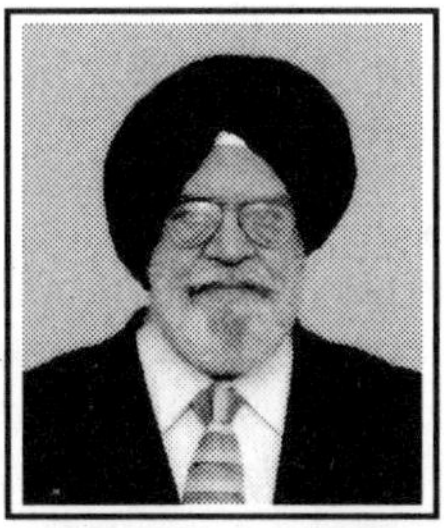

Prof. (Dr.) Jitendra Singh Bhatia
B.V.Sc & A.H., M.Sc. (A.I.I.M.S.) Ph.D.
Former ADG (Education, Development and Planning)
ICAR and Professor of Veterinary Physiology
Presently Professor and Head of Veterinary Physiology and Biochemistry,
Khalsa College of Veterinary and Annual Sciences, Amritsar-143 002

PREFACE

This book entitled 'A glimpse on Veterinary Education in India' has been planned as a referral document embodied therein some aspects of existing scenario that has been culminated through successive developments taken place ever since time immemorial. Further, based on the current ground status, some measures have been presented to make system more relevant in order to meet the existing challenges and future needs.

This book is a composite document with compilation of several of my articles/ write ups published/circulated and outcome of the experience and studies made during the recent past. It covers chapters on History of Veterinary Education in Indian Sub-continent, available resources pertinent to this sector, strategies for resource management, gap analysis and possible measures to bring reforms in overall growth of livestock sector. Some reflections toward Post Graduate (PG) education have also been covered. Education through private sector and feasibility to explore 'Public Private Partnership' in veterinary education has been attempted with the view to add new dimensions to educational set up. Possible approach in stream lining and managing lower education and continuing education programs has been suggested. Further, a chapter on regulatory and governance mechanisms in managing the affairs of veterinary educational system reflects my personal concepts and interpretations with no legal authentications.

It is very heartening to record my appreciations for the subject matter specialists who have been gracious in showering their wisdom by presenting write up on the vital issues relevant to veterinary educational trainings at TVCC, ILFC and Clinical diagnostics etc. It cannot be disputed that extension education in the broad umbrella of veterinary curriculum is weak in this sector and transfer of technological practices for the benefits of end users-the livestock farm community require a renewal approach. Extension educationists have consolidated their thoughts with their wide exposures and on field experiences by contributing a chapter on 'An ideal Approach to Extension Education in Veterinary University/Institution'.

In order to make a comprehensive document, relevant information have been picked up from various reports/documents/profiles/policy papers/annual reports/Acts, Statutes, Regulations/Guidelines/Publications of GOI, VCI, ICAR, universities, national academy, newsletters etc. Some useful information contained in these documents has been reproduced as such. Repetition at times became unavoidable so as to make a composite reading of a chapter.

The author has previlaged of having visited some of the universities/ colleges/institutes and drawn perceptions on the other institutions based on some reports/publications/personal contacts etc. Every possible care has been taken to present correct status as of now. However, some unrealistic reflections may have occurred in the document due to oversight or wrong perceptions. I may be excused if some comments are contrary to the present status of the institutes/ organizations/individuals.

I feel honored to express my gratefulness to Dr. Jit Singh, Dr. H.K. Verma, Dr. Jaswinder Singh Dr. Vishnu Sharma, Dr. (Mrs.) Sanjita Sharma, Dr. Adarsh Kumar, Dr. Ashok Srivastava and Dr. Manoj Kumar who have contributed chapters that have vital relevance to the professional developments.

The management of Khalsa College Charitable Society is profusely thanked for having permitted me to write this book. A special mention is made for Sardar Rajender Mohan Singh, Chhina, Honorary Secretary, Khalsa College Governing Council, who encouraged me to do this venture. He ensured proper support and encouragement in accomplishing this job. I will fail in my duty if I do not offer special thanks to Principal Khalsa college, Dr.S.K Jand and officiating Principal Dr.S.S.Sidhu both of whom have provided all the support and facilities in preparation of this document. Dr. S.K. Nagpal, Professor of veterinary anatomy is thanked for having shared my responsibilities during the time I was busy in preparation of this book.

This venture would not have been possible without the encouragement and guidance provided to me by Prof. Ajey Gahlot, VC, RAJUVAS, Bikaner and Prof. V.K. Taneja, VC, GADVASU with whom I continue to share my thoughts and their valuable advice offered from time to time has been handy to me in preparation of this book. Prof. M.P. Yadav, Secretary NAAS, and former Director of IVRI and VC, (SBBPUAT), Meerut, deserves all appreciation for having taken great pains to edit manuscript that has greatly helped me in shaping this book. I owe great appreciation to my wife Sardarni Satwant Kaur, who has been a pillar of strength during my entire professional career. Last but not the least; I am thankful to Sh.Rajwinder Singh who has helped me in typing this book.

Dr. Jitendra Singh Bhatia

ACRONYMS

AAS	Atomic absorption spectrophotometer
AAU	Assam agricultural university, Guwahati , Assam
AAU	Anand agricultural university, Anand, Gujarat
AB&G	Animal Breeding & Genetics
ACVM	Apollo college of veterinary medicine, Jaipur
AD	After death (traditional date after the death of Jesus' birth)
AH	Animal Husbandry
AICE- SRF	All India Central Examination for Senior Research Fellowship of ICAR
AIIMS	All India Institute of Medical Sciences, New Delhi
ARS	Agricultural Research Scientist
BAU	Bihar Agricultural University, Ranchi, Jharkhand
BC	Before Christ (traditional date before the birth of Jesus Christ)
BHU	Banaras Hindu University, Allahabad, UP
BOD	Biological Oxygen Demand Test Incubator (Low temperature controlled Incubator)
BOM	Board of Management
BSMA	Broad Subject Matter Area (ICAR)
BVC	Bombay Veterinary College, Mumbai
BVSc	Bachelor of Veterinary Science
BVSc&AH	Bachelor of Veterinary Science & Animal Husbandry
CADRAD	Centre for Animal Diseases Research and Diagnosis (IVRI)
CAS	Career Advancement Scheme
CAU	Central Agricultural University, Imphal
CSKHPKVV	Choudhary Saravan Kumar Himachal Pradesh Krishi Vishwa Videaylaya, Palampur, HP
CGKDVV	Chattisgarh Kamdhenu Vishwa Videyalaya, Chattisgarh, Raipur
CIF	Central Instrumentation Facilities

CT	Computed Tomography
CT Scan	Computer aided Tomography
CVE	Continuing Veterinary Education
DAHDF	Department of Animal Husbandry Dairying & Fisheries, GOI, New Delhi
DARE	Department of Agriculture Research & Education, ICAR, New Delhi
DU	Deemed to be University
ELISA	Enzyme Linked Immuno Sorbent Analysis
ERDDL	Eastern Region Disease Diagnosis Lab of IVRI, Kolkata
FICCI	Federation of Indian Chamber of Commerce & Industries
GADVASU	Guru Angad Dev Veterinary and Animal Science University, Ludhiana, Pb
GBPUAT	Govind Ballab Pant University of Agriculture and Technology, Pantnagar, Uttrakhand
GBVC	Graduate from Bihar/ Bombay/ Bengal Veterinary College
GDP	Gross Domestic Product
GER	Graduate Enrollment Ratio
GLP	Good Laboratory Practice
GMVC	Graduate of Madras Veterinary College
GOI	Government of India
HOD	Head of the Department
HPLC	High Performance Liquid Chromatography
HRD	Human Resource Development
IBL	Imperial Bacteriology Laboratory
ICAR	Indian Council of Agricultural Research
ICT	Information Communication and Technology
ILFC	Instructional Livestock Farm Complex
ISO	International Organization for Standardization
IAMR	Institute of Applied Manpower Research
IT	Information Technology
IVC Act	Indian Veterinary Council Act, 1984
IVRI	Indian Veterinary Research Institute, Izatnagar, Bareilly, UP
JAU	Junagarh Agricultural University, Junagarh, Gujarat

JRF	Junior Research Fellowship
KU	Kamdhenu University, Gandhi Nagar, Gujarat
KCVAS	Khalsa College of Veterinary and Animal Sciences, Amritsar
KUVAS	Kerala University of Veterinary and Animal Sciences, Pookode, Kerala
KVAFU	Karnataka University of Veterinary and Animal Science, Bidar, Karnataka
KVK	Krishi Vigyan Kendra
LEO	Livestock Extension Officer
LFP	Livestock Farm Practice
LPM	Livestock Production and Management
LPT	Livestock Product Technology
LS	Livestock
LUVAS	Lala Lajpat Rai University of Veterinary & Animal Sciences, Hisar, Harayana
MAFSU	Maharashtra Animal & Fishery Sciences University Nagpur, MS
MSc	Master of Science
MSHAE	Minimum Standards of Higher Agricultural Education-Education Division ICAR
MSVE	Minimum Standards of Veterinary Education-degree Course (BVSc&AH), Regulations of the VCI
MVSc	Master of Veterinary Science
NAARM	National Academy of Agricultural Research Management, Hyderabad
NADS	National Academy of Dairy Sciences
NARES	National Agricultural Research & Education System
NAU	Navsari Agicultural University, Navasari, Gujarat
NAVS	National Academy of Veterinary Sciences, New Delhi
NCA	National Commission on Agriculture
NDDB	National Dairy Development Board, Anand, Gujarat
NDRI	National Dairy Research Institute, Karnal
NDUAT	Narendra Dev University of Agricultural & Technology, Faizabad, UP
NDVSU	Nanaji Deshmukh Veterinary Sciences University, Jabalpur, MP

NERDDL	North East Region Disease Diagnosis Laboratory of IVRI, Guwahati
NGO	Non Government Organization
NKC	National Knowledge Commission
NRDDL	North Region Disease Diagnosis Laboratory of IVRI, Jalandhar, Pb
NSSO	National Sample Survey Office
OFD	On Farm Demonstration
OFT	On Farm Trail
OIE	Office of International des Epizooties: World Organization for Animal Heath, France
OUAT	Orrisa University of Agriculture and Technology
PCR	Polymerase Chain Reaction
PG	Post Graduate
PGIVAS	Post Graduate Institute of Veterinary and Animal Sciences, Akola, MS
PGIVER	Post Graduate Institute of Veterinary Education and Research, Jaipur, Rajasthan
PhD	Doctor of Philosophy
PPP	Public and Private Partnership
RAJUVAS	Rajasthan University of Veterinary and Animal Sciences, Bikaner, Rajasthan
RAU	Rajendra Agricultural University, Samastipur, Pusa, Bihar
RDDL	Regional Disease Diagnosis Laboratory
RKVY	Rasthrey Krishi Vikas Yogna
RRTC	Regional Research Training Centre
RVP	Registered Veterinary Practioner
SAU	State Agricultural University
SBBPUAT	Sardar Ballab Bhai Patel University of Agricultural & Technology, Meerut, UP
SKRAU	Swami Keshwanand Rajasthan Agricultural University , Bikaner, Rajasthan
SKAUST-J	Shere Kashmir Agricultural University of Science & Technology, Jammu, J&K
SKAUST-K	Shere Kashmir Agricultural University of Science & Technology, Srinagar, J&K

SOP	Standard Operative Procedure
SRDDL	Southern Region Disease Diagnosis Laboratory of IVRI, Banglore, Karnataka
SRF	Senior Research Fellowship
SVC	State Veterinary Council
SVU	State Veterinary University
SVVU	Sri Venkateswara Veterinary University, Triputi
TANUVAS	Tamil Nadu University of Veterinary and Animal Sciences, Chennai, TN
TVCC	Teaching Veterinary Clinical Complex
UG	Under Graduate
UGC	University Grant Commission
UMMB	Urea Molasses Mineral Blocks
UV	Ultra Violet
VCI	Veterinary Council of India, New Delhi
VUTRC	Veterinary University Training and Research Center-RAJUVAS
WBUAFS	West Bengal University of Animal & Fishery Sciences, Kolkata
WRDDL	Western Region Disease Diagnosis Laboratory of IVRI, Pune, MS

CONTENTS

PART-I
Author's Perceptions (Composite Documentation on Various Facets of Veterinary Education)

PART-II
Invited Articles

PART-III
Abstracted Report, Reference, Publications and Articles having relevance to Veterinary Education

Part-I
Author's Perceptions-
Composite
Documentation
on Various Facets
of Veterinary Education

Chapter-1

Veterinary Education in India Historical Perspective

This chapter deals with successive developments of veterinary education since the period of human civilization, ancient period, modern period, veterinary institutions during pre-independent period, progressive growth during early post independent phase, vital transformations on introduction of land grant system of education, creation of regulatory authority- the VCI, establishment of veterinary and animal sciences universities and status of the institutions as of now.

1.1 Introduction

Veterinary education in Indian subcontinent is as old as human civilization here. Study of history of veterinary education will retell the political, ideological, religious and philosophical changes in the civilization in India.

The Aryans were primarily pastorals. Unlike the urban agricultural civilization of Indus-Valley and their very livelihood depended on cattle rearing. Aryans when settled around riverine Northern India (circa 2400 to 1500 BC), became agrarian tribes depending solely on agriculture and livestock for their livelihood. They appreciated the importance of livestock and in fact, the cattle became not only a source of their sustenance but formed their wealth. Cattle were most prized possession and inter-tribal wars were fought for acquiring cows (the term used was Govisthi or search for cows). Cows were symbol of wealth and status. Religion became closely associated with animals; hence cow became sacred. In Vedic literature cow, bull or ox are mentioned more frequently than any other spices of animal. Rig Veda which is considered to be the oldest written document, mentions about cattle. The main interest in cow formed a basis for the development of socio-economic life in India, which forms the structural backbone of Indian society. In fact, human civilization in ancient India has been considered to be based on cattle husbandry/culture.

Worldwide animals provided food, wealth, draft power, fiber, manure companionship as well considered symbol of prestige to people especially from affluent society. Animals were used as custodian of territory in war and peace and used extensively in tracking and expeditions. Animal husbandry practices remained an art until 18th century when first army school was established in 1827 at Pune. Subsequently the first civil veterinary educational school was opened at Lahore in 1882. However, when situation is viewed in context of global perspective of modern veterinary education, the very first veterinary school was established in Lyon in 1761 and thereafter at Alford, France in 1764. These became possible only through hectic persuasion of a French Veterinarian Claude Burgelet with King Louis XVI for creation of veterinary institutions. Some global developments taken place during that time and thereafter were.

England

1791 - Establishment of First Veterinary School in London

1823 - Establishment of Edinburgh Veterinary College in UK

USA

1852 - First Veterinary College Philadelphia created

1854 - Veterinary College New York was established

Canada

1862 - Opened Ontario Veterinary College which was later shifted to Guelph Ontario during 1922

Indian Sub-continent - Establishment of Veterinary Schools

1882 - First Punjab Veterinary School at Lahore (erstwhile united Punjab)

1886 - Second Veterinary School at Bombay

1893 - Third Veterinary School at Calcutta (now Kolkota) WB

1903 - Forth Veterinary School at Madras

1.2 Progressive Developments in Indian sub-continent

For the purpose of presenting sequential developments of this sector in Indian sub-continent, historical perspective is classified in three periods- Ancient, Medieval and Modern period.

1.2.1 Ancient Period

The Veterinary Education was endemic then and existed as a culture that was passed on from generation to generation through the word of mouth. Ancient period in chronological order is sub-divided as under :

1.2.1.1 Vedic Period: (Circa 1800 or 1500-1200 BC): Brahma one of the supreme cosmic diety, through human mediators is thought to have created the Veda as an ethical guide to the civilization. According to Hindu mythology, God Brahma composed Atharvaveda of which Ayurveda was a section dealing with knowledge of medicine. Gavya Ayurveda dealt with cattle and Hasti Ayurveda dealt with elephants. Elephants were used in wars like modern tanks by the kings in ancient India.

1.2.1.2 Epic Period: It is the period of Ramayana and Mahabharata. Some names and their works of this period include:

1. Salihotra wrote A svayureveda Siddayoga Samgraha, that is a treatise on horses. Some portions of original text are available along with its English, Arabic and Tibetan translations. Salihotras period was more or less fell during Pre-Puranic phase. Salihotra is said to have lived in Salutar, a country near Gandhara the modern Kandahar. Some place him to Taksila.
2. Palakapya, Probably contemporary of Salihotra, wrote Hasthyayurveda, that is a treatise on elephants.
3. Nakula (youngst of Pandov brother) wrote A'sva Cikitsa, that is treatment of horses; Vaidyaka Sarvasva, that is documentation on medicines.
4. Sahadeva (elder to Nakul) wrote Vyadhisindhu Vimardana, that is the cure of ocean of diseases. He was an expert of cattle and is understood to have authored a book on cattle named as Gosastra.

1.2.1.3 Puranic period: This period probably was between Epic and Mauryan period. The several puranas in which informations on veterinary interest are available include Matsya purana, Agni purana,

Brahmanda purana, Vishnu purana and Linga purana. Vishnu purana and Matsya purana describes the criteria for selection of the bulls for breeding purpose (an equivalent of it is Panchyati bull still prevalent in Haryana and some other states).

1.2.1.4 Mauryan period: (324 to 187 BC) Chanakya is known to have authored Kautilya-Artha'sastra that contains valuable information on animal husbandry practices.

1.2.1.5 Manu's period: (circa 200 BC-200 AD) Manu Samhita has descriptions about animal husbandry.

1.2.1.6 Artha'sastra of Post-Vedic period gives the detailed account of administration, functionaries, responsibilities, wages, feeding, breeding and cruelty about animals. It was during the period of King Ashok's regime, hundreds of well equipped veterinary hospitals were established. Each hospital was headed by a Salihotra who was paid by the government. Even during the Raj era, the veterinarian in Northern India was called as 'Salutri, the etymology of which can lead us to Salihotriya. These were the first veterinary hospitals known world over. Herbs were used as healing medicines.

In ancient India the population of each tribe was small and inhabitants were so closely related that they needed no formal administration. Moreover, acquisition of knowledge was complicated and restricted to a few. One could become a veterinarian by working with the teacher at his dwelling or gurukul.

The Ayurvedic school of medicine went in the antiquity due to predominance of Buddhism and invasion of Ancient Greek or Greeco-Arabic school of medicine (Unani). The contemporary of Ayurvedic practice was Greek School of medicine. Among Greeks, Hippocrates (460-370 BC) used to teach extensively about fractures, dislocations and wound treatment. The classical Greek period is described as an important era in the development of human medicine. The medical practice of ancient Greece is actually the precursor of the present day Western medical practice or Allopathic school of medicine.

Nearly up to 1000 AD there was no major development in medicine. Medical knowledge of these civilizations received set back due to supremacy of Islamic culture in Middle East and partly in Europe, rapid spread of Christianity in most of the Western Countries and probably dominance of Buddhism in Indian continent. Dominance of religion neglected the development of science as it preached philosophy that believed, the diseases were punishment by GOD or celestial bodies for evil deeds. Greeks had medical knowledge from Egyptians. It then spread to other Western and Arabian Countries. Arabs learned surgical craft and knowledge of medicine from Nestorians. Nestorian was a persecuted Christian sect which sought refuge in the deserts, where they came in contact with Arab tribes. The Greek and Roman medical texts were translated in to Arabic at that time. In Western countries when Christians became liberal, they created modern Allopathic School of Medicine and with Muslims in Middle Eastern and Asian countries it developed Unani School of medicine.

1.2.2 Medieval Period (1206-1761 AD)

So far as the Mogul period is concerned, Ain-i-Akbari by Abu-L-Fazal, which gives history during Akbar ruling till 1602, is an important source for animal husbandry, and it, in fact, in considered of same value for medieval India as Kautilya,s Arthasastra is considered for ancient India. The Ain-i-Akbari provides information on breeding and feeding of elephants, horses, mules, camels and cows.

1.2.3 Modern Period

Under British rule, the Indian educational system was initially ignored. It was much later that the British deliberately decided to suppress the indigenous system. In nineteenth century British Government surveyed the Indian educational system that was in shambles. And it was their opportunism to reorganize it to suit their needs. In 1823, Raja Ram Mohan Roy beseeched the British Government not to deny modern education to Indians. More liberal and enlightened system of instruction was promoted, and seed of the then modern system of education found its place in Indian soil. Schools and colleges came in to existence and in 1857 three universities- The Madras, Bombay and Calcutta Universities came in to existence. These were different from mere oriental education through Islamic Madrasas and Sanskrit Pathshalas. British ignored the fact that education is the slow process of growth adapting to the needs of the country and culture. They wanted Indians to be literate enough to make their administration smooth and easy.

1.3 Veterinary Training and Education-structural developments

1.3.1 Training institutions

Beginning from 1000 AD there was total eclipse of veterinary science in India till 18th century when East India Company became interested in improving the quality of horses and bullocks for military purposes. Lt. William Frazer was entrusted the job of establishing a stud farm at Pusa Bihar for improving horse breeding in 1795. Later, William Moorcraft (1799), the first western veterinarian was called to improve the condition of Pusa stud which was not making the desired progress. He was able to provide better strategy for feeding, breeding and disease management. William Moorcraft is considered as the first qualified veterinarian to arrive in India.

In order to have more personnel trained in the than modern veterinary and animal husbandry practices, the first training course on veterinary sciences was organized in 1821 by J.T. Hodgson. This had shown the seed of allopathic school of veterinary medicine which is now flourishing in India. Britishers established their first Army Veterinary Department at Poona in 1827, to cater the then increasing need of horses. With time in 1862, an Army Veterinary School was also established in Poona. Their main thrust was breeding, nutrition and management of horses required for the army. During the time Indian cattle suffered a severe outbreak of plague (Rinderpest) which greatly affected the Indian agriculture operations and food production. This led to the establishment of Indian Plague Commission in 1869. Colonel J.B. Hallen who acted as chairman of the commission recommended that proper veterinary training should be organized to tackle problems of diseases of livestock in future. Civil Veterinary Department was also established. Colonel J.B. Hallen also acted its first Inspector General. Madras - the first state where veterinary training establishment was set up. With this, Britishers started showing their interest in cattle for improving production and transport. In furtherance to their main concern for horses, they went to the extent of utilizing services (from around 1872) onward at already established equine breeding farm (EBS) spread in 2039 acres at Babugarh in 1811 at Uttar Pradesh (then United Provinces) for practical instruction in management of horses in stables, and cultivation of fodder crops for them. The Government of India had realized that horse and mule breeding operations took up so much of the veterinary officers' time that cattle breeding and control of diseases have suffered a severe set-back. The teaching program on equines thus was discontinued after two years.

Subsequently some more Army Veterinary Schools were opened, that is at Hapur in 1877, Ajmer in 1881 and Shimla in 1888. The schools at Ajmer and Shimla existed for very short period. The Army Veterinary School at Hapur (not to confuse with Army Stud at Babugarh) was also closed in 1882 and the students were shifted to Punjab Veterinary School - Lahore (now in Pakistan), where the first ever civil veterinary school (that still continue to exist) in the Colonial India was established. Ajmer School, vide supra, was also closed in 1905 and its mobile assets along with students were also shifted to Punjab Veterinary College Lahore.

A Bacteriological lab established at Poona in 1889 was later shifted to Mukteshwar in Kumaon hills of Dist. Naniital as Imperial Bacteriological Lab and then re-designated as Imperial Institute of Veterinary Research and presently has become a multi campus organization- the Indian Veterinary Research Institute (IVRI) with main campus at Izatnagar.

1.3.2 Establishment of Veterinary Educational Institutions

1.3.2.1 Pre-partition period

The Punjab Veterinary School was the first non-military educational instruction that started in 1882 with the then modern system of medicine i.e. allopathic system is a formal way - (Fig-1) A two year "Veterinary Assistant" Course was started with Urdu as medium of instruction. Soon thereon it started LVP (Licentiate in Veterinary Practice sing certification). Subsequently, a veterinary college (BVC) was started in Bombay in 1886- (Fig-2) The Bengal Veterinary School (BVC) at Calcutta in 1893 and Madras Veterinary College (MVC) came in existence in 1903. The Veterinary education was further extended by opening Bihar

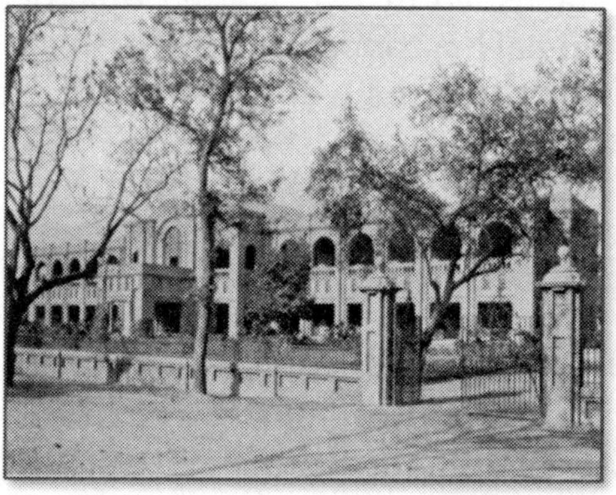

Fig. 1 : First Veterinary College in Undivided INDIA, Lahore

Veterinary College at Patna in 1927. These collages awarded Diplomas to their graduates that were known by the names of the States, viz., GBVC i.e. Graduate of Bombay/ Bengal/ Bihar Veterinary Colleges; GMVC i.e. Graduate of Madras Veterinary College.

A course leading to the degree of 'Bachelor of Veterinary Sciences' (B.V.Sc) was introduced at the Madras Veterinary College in 1936, and since then other institutions followed this example. The Last institution before partition was the establishment of Government Veterinary College at Hyderabad in 1946.

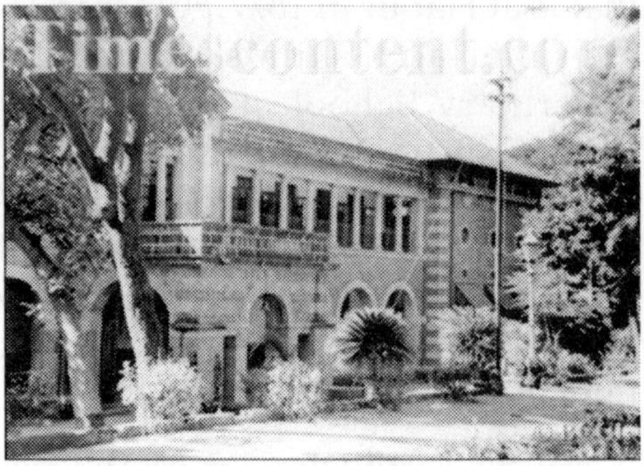

Fig. 2 : Bombay Veterinary College, Mumbai

In 1942 the Punjab Veterinary College was affiliated to the Punjab University and a four and a half year degree course of B.V.Sc was started, while retaining matriculation as the entry level qualification. In due course of time, these colleges were affiliated to the general universities in the regions and full-fledged degree program on traditional annual system of education came in existence. The Mathura Veterinary College established in 1947 started dual degree course by incorporation 37% Animal husbandry segements in the course contents and the graduates were conferred with BVSc & AH degree. Soon other colleges followed suit by modifying course contents making room for animal husbandry subjects in the degree course. All colleges other than Madras started conferring BVSc&AH degree while MVC retained degree nomenclature of BVSc.

1.3.2.2 Post partition phase

In 1947 the political scenario of the Indian sub-continent changed. Along with the transmigration of people between newly formed India and Pakistan, Indian students and teachers from Punjab Veterinary College were shifted to Hisar. The Veterinary College of Hisar is outcome of bifurcated Punjab Veterinary College, Lahore, at the time of partition in 1947. With the help of the then migrated staff from Lahore Veterinary College, the Punjab Government set up a Camp Veterinary College in a government school premises. The college at Hisar started functioning from February 15, 1948.

To meet the growing needs of livestock sector and prioritization of the country to strengthen rural developmental programs, 9 more colleges were added by 1960 thereby raising the number to 15. All the colleges were State animal husbandry controlled organizations offering 4 years degree course of BVSc&AH following British pattern of traditional education.

1.3.2.3 Structural reforms in agricultural education-by GOI

Without loss of any time soon after independence, Govt. of India appointed the Indian University Education Commission in 1948, with Dr Sarvapalli Radhakrishan, the then Vice President of India as its chairman (later he became second President of India). The commission had not only expanded the scope of the term of reference of the committee by adding agricultural education to the expanding spectrum of education but also kept agriculture on the top of its agenda so as to speedily reduce the drudgeries of farming community and enable them to get better manage mental and advisory services to boost farm and Livestock productivity to pull out India out of food crisis so as to make India 'self sufficient' and 'self reliant' in food front.

A concept 'Rural Universities' (different from the land grant system) was mooted by Dr. S. Radha Krishnan commission. The agricultural education transformed into a new shape after a separate education system (trimester system with total internal evaluation) in agriculture was suggested by the Joint Indo-American Team of Agricultural Research and Education in 1955 (Mr Damle as Chairman). Later on in 1960 the second Joint Indo-American Team (DR N.S. Randhawa as Chairman) recommended that;

- Granting autonomous status to the institutions
- Agriculture, Veterinary, Home science, Technology in Agricultural Sciences at all campuses
- Integration of teaching of different faculties
- Integration of teaching research and extension education

1.3.2.4 Establishing State Agricultural Universities

In 1960, Ralph W. Cumming, field Director, Rockefeller, advised State Governments on legislation for Agricultural universities and soon thereafter, the first agricultural university was inaugurated by Pandit Jawahar Lal Nehru the first Prime Minister of India in 1960 at

Pantnagar at the foot hills of Himalayas, UP (now in Uttrakhand). Soon many more States had created Agricultural Universities. All the existing Veterinary Colleges until that time and those created thereafter become constituent units of State Agricultural Universities (SAUs). These Colleges being constituent units of SAUs, their management, growth and governance were linked with the university development policies and programs.

All agricultural universities have been created in a State through enactment of Legislative Act of the respective State. Soon the Indian Council of Agricultural Research (ICAR) took the onus to aid, promote, regulate and integrate agricultural universities. To bring uniformities in governance system between the universities, the ICAR created a Model Act in 1966 (lately revised in 2009). This Act became a guiding force for the agricultural universities to function. All SAU's created thereafter were legislated primarily on the basis of ICAR Model Act. The claim of the ICAR as apex organization was strengthened by the cabinet decision (1973) to entrust responsibilities to the Department of Agricultural Research and Education (DARE) of coordinating agricultural education in the country, as ICAR has already been discharging the function which is equivalent to UGC in matter of regulating agricultural education.

Another landmark decision of the ICAR was to constitute the First Dean's Committee in 1971. The term of reference for this committee was primarily to update course curricula and academic regulations for all the faculties of agricultural education. The ICAR made it mandatory for SAU's to follow the recommendations of Dean's committee in their universities. Second Deans committee (1981-85) in its report streamlined the academic regulations, credit course requirements under trimester/ semester plans and recommended increase in degree duration by making mandatory requirements of 6 calendar month of internship for BVSc&AH degree requirement. Two more Dean's committees were constituted (third and fourth) in 1994 and 2006. Development Grant of the ICAR for strengthening education was linked with the adoption of Dean's committee recommendations. This has enpowered the ICAR to implement its policies and programs in SAU's more effectively. First two Dean's committees had revised and updated veterinary educational programs and subsequently this function was entrusted to the Veterinary Council of India (VCI) through statutory authority granted to it by virtue of promulgation of IVC Act, 1984.

1.3.2.5 Promulgation of Indian Veterinary Council Act (IVC Act)

The National Commission on Agriculture ((NCA) in a report stated that during pre-independence days only the Veterinarians qualifying from the Royal Veterinary College in the United Kingdom registered under the Veterinary Surgeons Act-1881 were legally authorized in India to issue professional certificate such as those for legal cases, import and export of livestock and livestock products etc. The Veterinarians qualifying from the Veterinary colleges of our country did not have such legal authority as there was no statutory recognized body either at the centre or in most of the states for their registration. The practice is still in vogue in case of import and export of race horses. In December, 1951 at a joint meeting of the All India Veterinary Association and Bombay Veterinary Medical Association under the chairmanship of the then Union Minister of Food and Agriculture, this matter surfaced. The Minister appointed a Steering Committee to go in to the question of establishing a National Veterinary Council. In due course of time the Steering Committee recommended that;

1. State Veterinary Councils be set up by a legislature in the States on the model of the Utter Pradesh Veterinary Council Act - 1947.
2. A statutory Veterinary Council of India be set up by providing representation on this body from the State Councils to
   a) Provide a statutory organization representing the veterinary profession to serve as a liaison body between the Government of India and the International Veterinary Congress.
   b) Control and regulate the practice of the profession and the conduct of its members and to uphold the status and dignity of the profession.
   c) Arrange for reciprocity of the various veterinary qualifications in inter-state and international circles.
   d) Maintain a recognized Register of Veterinary Practitioners in the country and to give evidence as an expert under Section-45 of the Indian Evidence Act on any matter pertaining to the veterinary profession.

The Government of India, Ministry of Agriculture on the recommendations made by the National Commission of Agriculture, during the early part of the Sixth Plan period introduced a bill in the Parliament entitled, "The Indian Veterinary Council Bill-1981" and consequent upon the passing of the bill, the Indian Veterinary Council

Act was enacted in 1984. It received the assent of the President of Republic of India on August 18, 1984 and published by the Ministry of Law, Justice and Company Affairs (Legislative Department), for general information in the Gazette of India (Extraordinary, Part-II, Section-1); No.52; New Delhi, Tuesday, August 21, 1984. It envisaged the establishment of the Veterinary Council of India (VCI) at the Centre and State Veterinary Councils (SVC) in such States and Union Territories which have/had adopted the Indian Veterinary Council Act.

1.3.2.6 Creation of the Veterinary Council of India (VCI)

The Ministry of Agriculture, Government of India exercised the powers conferred by subsection-1, section-3, chapter-II of the Indian Veterinary Council Act - 1984; and constituted a statutory body the 'Veterinary Council of India' by nominating twenty seven members of the council vide Gazette notification of August 2, 1989.

The Veterinary Council of India in its first meeting held on January 12, 1990, unanimously elected Dr C.M. Singh and Dr. R.P.S Tyagi as President and Vice President, respectively and seven members of Executive Committee of the Council.

1.3.2.7 Determination of 'Minimum Standards of Veterinary Education-Degree course (BVSc&AH) Regulations' (MSVE)

The Veterinary Council of India (VCI) a statutory authority was created to regulate Veterinary Practice in the country. The said IVC Act under section 22 empowered the VCI to prescribe 'Minimum Standards of Veterinary Education- degree course (BVSc&AH)' Regulations, (MSVE). The VCI laid down MSVE, Regulations in 1993 which primarily pertains to;

1. Academic regulation pertaining to eligibility qualification, admission procedure, duration of degree course, examination and evaluation, passing percentage.
2. Syllabus, course curriculum and credit distribution
3. Minimum requirement pertaining to buildings, departments, staff (Teaching and supporting), equipment and other support system.

The Veterinary Council of India took mammoth exercise to revamp MSVE Regulation, 1993. New regulations have been brought out in 2008. A reasonably good attempt was made by the VCI to :

1. Update the syllabus and redistribution of course credit.
2. Greater emphasis on' Hands on Training' by incorporating non credit courses on;
   - Entrepreneurial development
   - Tracking courses
   - Study circle
3. Internship program has been made meaningful and linked to acquisition of minimum core competence skills (Part V (6) of MSVE, Regulation, 2008).
4. Manpower requirements have been made more realistic.
5. Infrastructure needs updated with newer technological innovations and scientific developments.
6. Establishing Instructional Livestock Farm Complex ILFC-a mandatory requirement.

The Veterinary Colleges continued to be components of SAU's and were/are being aided supported by ICAR. However, to regulate standards of veterinary education for degree course, VCI took over the control in those states where the IVC Act, 1984 has been extended. Despite the fact that VCI is the statutory authority to regulate veterinary education, it is yet to put in place regulations for PG education. The ICAR through its accreditation board has brought structural changes to master's and doctorate programs for veterinary education in 2006. These new guidelines have been implemented in all veterinary institutions. Thus presently VCI is only regulating the degree course while ICAR is aiding for UG & PG educational programs and regulating PG education at veterinary institutions.

1.3.2.8 Establishment of Veterinary Universities

The first Veterinary University was established at Chennai (Tamil Nadu) in 1989 by carving out veterinary, animal sciences, dairy and fisheries components from the existing Tamil Nadu Agricultural University, Coimbatore. The basic organizational structure, governance pattern and academic pattern of State Agricultural Universities (SAUs) were retained by the newly created Veterinary University.

During the last century two more veterinary universities came into being, the first at West Bengal in 1995 and another at Maharashtra

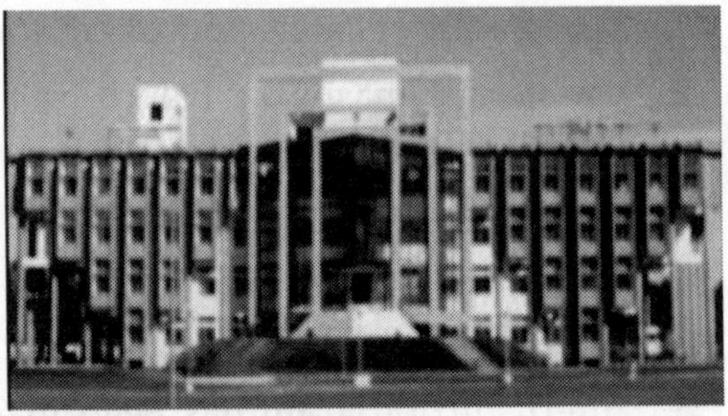

Fig. 3 : First Veterinary University in India, TANUVAS, Chennai,1989

in 2000. In a span of first 10 years of 21st century, 10 more universities have been established in Punjab, UP, AP, Karnataka, Rajasthan, Haryana, MP, Kerala, Chhattisgarh and Gujarat. The Kamdhenu Veterinary University created at Gujarat is yet to establish a veterinary college. With the creation of Veterinary Universities, Veterinary Colleges became constituent units of these universities except in the State of Gujarat where none of the 4 existing veterinary colleges attached to SAU's have been transferred to the State's own Veterinary University (SVU). Of the Total 46 constituent veterinary colleges in the country, 2/3 colleges are the constituents unit of SVU's. Leaving one Govt. veterinary college at Puducherry, rest of the Veterinary Colleges are constituent units of SAUs.

1.3.2.9 Education through Private Sector

Privatization of veterinary education has added new dimensions to this professional set up with the creation of first private Veterinary College in 2003-the Apollo College of Veterinary Medicine (ACVM) at Jaipur, Rajasthan. Today there are 7 private colleges in Rajasthan, one each in Punjab and UP. Haryana has already been accorded permission to open colleges in the state which has become operational during 2014-15 academic session.

1.3.2.10 Education in Animal Sciences from Agricultural Universities/ Colleges

PG courses in various disciplines of animal sciences are also offered by the agricultural colleges. Many agricultural colleges in private sector are offering PG education in animal/dairy/poultry sciences. There is no regulatory control over these programs. It is unfortunate that some of these colleges are offering sub-standard education. The VCI and the ICAR must take stock of the situation and ensure that no non-accredited program should operate in the country.

1.4 Present Status of Veterinary educational institutions

Presently there are over 60 veterinary colleges in India (Table 1). Among these, 32 are part of veterinary (inclusive of animal and fishery Science) universities. Fourteen of SAUs are having 15 constituent colleges. While the veterinary college at Aizwal in Mizoram is a constituent college of Central Agricultural University (CAU) in Imphal, the veterinary college at Pundacherry is affiliated to general University of Pundacherry. A number of states have more than one veterinary college. Amongst these Rajasthan, Maharashtra, Andhra Pradesh, Karnataka, Gujarat, Tamil Nadu, Madhya Pradesh and Uttar Pradesh have 9,6,5,4,4,4, 3, and 3 veterinary colleges, respectively. Rest of the States has one or two colleges, generally corresponding to the number of SAUs.

Table 1 : Distribution of Veterinary Colleges in India. (Enlistment of insitution is seen at Annexure-I)

Constituent Colleges: 50		
(i)	State Veterinary Universities (SVU)	32
(ii)	State Agriculture Universities (SAU)	15
(iii)	Central Agricultural University (CAU)	01
(iv)	Central General University	01
Affiliated Colleges: 11		
(i)	Government Veterinary College	01
(ii)	Private Veterinary Colleges	10
	Total	**60**

Further, out of the 3 Deemed Universities (DUs) under ICAR, dealing with veterinary, animal science and/ or fishery science education, IVRI, Izatnagar offers master's and doctoral programs in almost all branches of veterinary and animal sciences. Similarly NDRI, Karnal offers higher educational programs in dairy science, dairy technology and dairy husbandry, both at undergraduate and postgraduate levels. CIFE, Mumbai is offering educational programs in fishery sciences.

In nutshell, it may sound good that the professional institutional network has grown 10 fold after independence (from 6 to 60) and India has more than double the number of Veterinary education institutions than the second next being USA having 28 colleges. However, numerically our system have not grown in commen-

suration with the diversification that has taken place over the time. With ever increasing societal dependency and challenges surmounting, an aggressive approach is needed not only to cover up the short falls but to build institutions of the order that are able to deliver effectively in meeting expected social needs.

Land mark (Dates) decisions relevant to Veterinary education

18th Century

1. 1795 - Lt William Frezer, a non veterinarian, entrusted to establish stud farm near PUSA.
2. 1799 - William Moorcraft, the first western veterinarian called to improve conditions of Pusa Stud farm.

19th Century

3. 1821 - JT Hodgson organized training centre on modern veterinary and AH practices. It made a beginning of Allopathic School.
4. 1827 - First Army Veterinary Department established at Pune.
5. 1862 - Army school established in Pune. Subsequently some more army schools opened. A school established in 1877 at Ajmer but then closed in 1882 and students were shifted to Punjab Veterinary School, Lahore.
6. 1869 - Owing to serve outbreak of cattle Plague (Rinderpest), Indian Cattle Plague Commission established under the chairmanship of Col. J. B. Heller. Col. Hellnen was also appointed as first Inspector General at Madras. Madras was the first State where animal training establishment set up.

Establishment of Veterinary Educational Institutions

7. 1882 - Punjab Veterinary school Lahore- First non-military educational institution established. The Colleges at Bombay-1886, Madras- 1903, Patna- 1927 and Andhra Pradesh- 1946 followed subsequently.
8. 1889 - Imperial Bacteriological Laboratory (IBL) established at Poona was later shifted to Mukteshwar in Kumaon

hills and re-designated as Imperial Institute of Veterinary Research, presently a multi campus organization- the Indian Veterinary Research Institute (IVRI) with the main campus at Izatnagar. Though, Post graduate college at IVRI was established in 1958 with its affiliation with Agra University and on later date with Rohilkhand in 1975 but it finally got 'Deemed to be University' status by UGC in 1983.

9. 1936 - Madras veterinary college was first to introduce BVSc degree course other followed subsequently. Entry level qualification for the degree course continued to be Matric.

Post Independence Era

10. 1947 1948 - Veterinary Colleges at Mathura, Hisar, Jabalpur and Assam created. College at Hisar has been the outcome of bifurcation of Punjab Veterinary College, Lahore.

11. 1948 - Indian Education Commission appointed under chairmanship of Dr. Sarvapalli Radhakridhnan. The commission stressed the need for strengthening agricultural education. It also coined the concept of RURAL UNIVERSITIES.

12. 1955 - First joint Indo American Team of Agricultural Education constituted under Mr. Damle.

13. 1960 - Second joint Indo American Team constituted under Dr. N. S. Randhawa.

14. 1960 - First Agricultural University created at Pantnagar as per US model of Land Grant System of Education. Veterinary College was one of the constituent units of this University.

15. 1966 - ICAR created model Act- A guiding principle for establishment of SAUs. Lately revised in 2009.

16. 1971 - First Dean's Committee Constituted by ICAR.

17. 1973 - Cabinet entrusted the responsibilities to department of Agriculture Research and Education (DARE) to coordinate agricultural education in the country.

18. 1981 - Second, third (1995) and fourth (2004) Dean's Committees Constituted by ICAR. Fifth Dean's committee is presently working.

19. 1984 - IVC Act 1984 promulgated.

20. 1989 - VCI constituted under the provision of IVC Act 1984.

21. 1989 - First Veterinary and Animal Sciences University created as Madras.

22. 1991 - GOI issued notification for establishment of a separate department of Animal Husbandry and Dairying under Ministry of Agriculture (Gazette of India Extraordinary para-2 Section (iii) sub-section (ii).

23. 1993 - National Academy of Veterinary Sciences registered with the Registrar of Societies.

24. 1993 - VCI laid down Minimum Standard of Veterinary Education-degree course (BVSc A.H), Regulations.

25. 2003 - First veterinary college under private sector at Jaipur, (Rajasthan) established.

26. 2005 - Status report on Veterinary Colleges in India- A study made by the VCI.

27. 2008 - Veterinary Council of India- VCI organized National Seminar at Hyderabad.

28. 2009 - Constitution of the Balaraman Committee to examine manpower requirement of Veterinary Colleges offering only UG education.

29. 2013 - Report of expert Committee on education constitution by Central Government.

30. 2013 - NAVS workshop on veterinary education on human resources needs in Animal Husbandry sector at Jaipur, Rajasthan.

31. 2014 - ICAR constituted a committee to determine minimum standards of Higher Veterinary Education (MSHVE).

VETERINARY UNIVERSITES IN INDIA

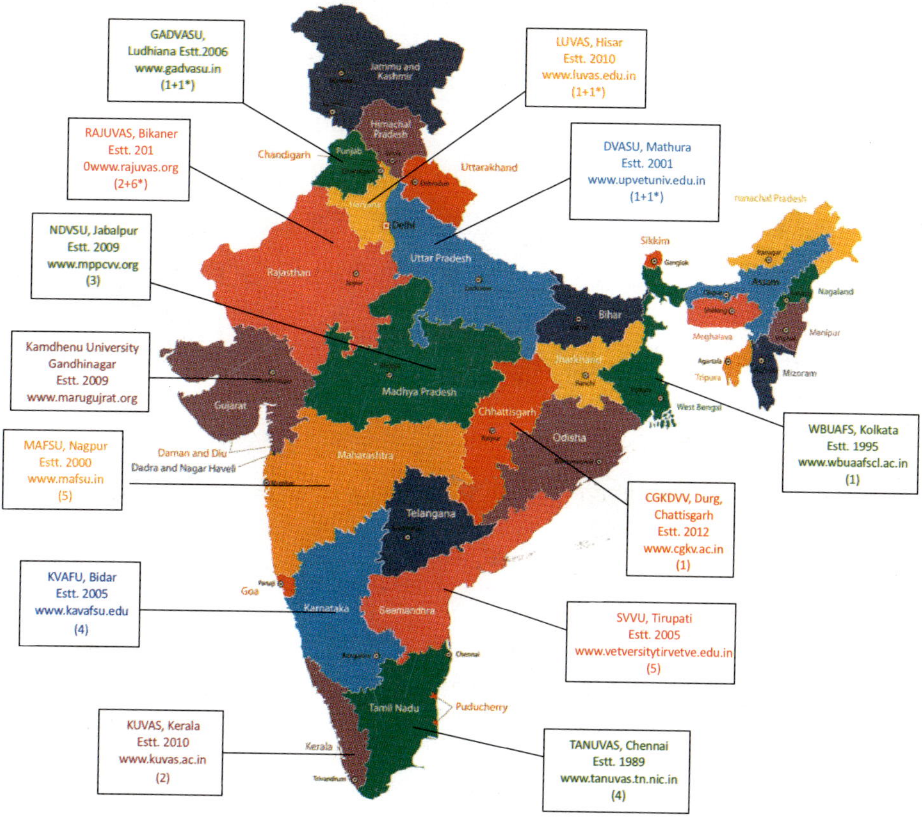

PG Colleges
1. PGIVAS, (MAFSU) Akola, MS
2. PGIVER,(RAJUVAS) Jaipur, RAJ
3. IVRI, IZZATNAGAR, Barielly, UP

( ) denote number of Colleges
* Private College

ANNEXURE-1

VETERINARY EDUCATIONAL INSTITUTIONS IN INDIA

A. Veterinary Universities and constituent colleges in INDIA

I. Tamil Nadu University of Veterinary and Sciences (TANUVAS)-TAMIL NADU (1989)

1. Madras Veterinary College, Chennai, TN (1903)
2. Veterinary College & Research Institute, Namakkal, TN (1986)
3. Veterinary College Orathanadu*, TN (2011)
4. Veterinary College & Research Institute, Tirunelveli*, TN (2011)

II. West Bengal University of Animal and Fisheries Sciences (WBUAFSC)-WB (1995)

5. Faculty of Veterinary Science, Kolkata, WB (1893)

III. Maharashtra Animal and Fisheries Science University (MAFSU)–NAGPUR, MS (2000)

6. Bombay Veterinary College, Parel, Mumbai (1886)
7. Nagpur Veterinary College, Nagpur (1958)
8. College of Veterinary and Animal Sciences, Parbhani (1972)
9. College of Veterinary Science, Udgir, Distt. Latur *(1987)
10. KNP College of Veterinary and Animal Sciences, Shirwal*, Satara (1988)
11. PG Institute of Veterinary Science, Akola* (1970)

IV. Deen Dayal Upadhaya Pasu Vigyan awam Go- Anusandhan Sansthan (DUVASU) MATHURA, UP (2001)

12. College of Veterinary Science & Animal Husbandry, Mathura (1947)

V. Karnataka Veterinary, Animal and Fisheries Science University (KVAFU)-BIDAR, KARNATAKA (2005)

13. Veterinary College Hebbel, Bangaluru, Karnataka (1959)
14. Veterinary College Nandinagar, Bidar, Karnataka (1984)
15. Veterinary Colloge, Shivamogga*, Karnataka (2008)

16. Veterinary Collage, Hasan*, Karnataka (2009)

VI. Sri Venkateswara Veterinary University (SVVU)-TIRUPATI, AP (2005)

17. College of Veterinary Science, Hyderabad (1946)

18. College of Veterinary Science, Tirupati (1955)

19. N,T.R College of Veterinary Science, Gannavaram (1997)

20. College of Veterinary Science, Korutla* (2008)

21. College of Veterinary Science, Proddatur* (2009)

VII. Guru Angad Dev Veterinary and Animal Science University (GADVASU)-LUDHIANA, PUNJAB (2006)

22. College of Veterinary Science, Ludhiana (1969)

VIII. Nanaji Deshmukh Veterinary Science University (NDVSU)-JABALPUR, MP (2009)

23. College of Veterinary Science & Animal Husbandry,Jabalpur (1948)

24. College of Veterinary Science & Animal Husbandry, Mhow (1956)

25. College of Veterinary Science, Rewa* (2007)

IX. Rajasthan University of Veterinary and Animal Sciences (RAJUVAS)-BIKANER, RAJASTHAN (2010)

26. College of Veterinary Science Animal Husbandry, Bikaner (1954)

27. College of Veterinary and Animal Science, Navania* Udaipur (2007)

28. PG Institue of Veterinary Education & Research (PGIVER), Jaipur (2012)

X. Lala Lajpat Rai University of Veterinary and Animal Sciences (LUVAS)-HISAR, HARYANA (2010)

29. College of Veterinary Sciences, Hisar (1948)

XI. Kerala Veterinary and Animal Sciences University (KUVAS)-POOKODE, KERALA (2010)

30. College of Veterinary and Animal Science,Mannuthy (1955)
31. College of Veterinary and Animal Science, Pookode* (2004)

XII. Chattisgarh Kamdhenu Viswa Vidayalya (CGKDVV)- ANJORA, DURG, CHATTISGARH (2012)

32. College of Veterinary Science & Animal Hsbandry, Durg (1985)

B. Veterinary colleges with State Agricultural Universities (SAUs)

33. College of Veterinary Science & Animal Husbandry, Anand, Gujarat (AAU) 1964
34. Faculty of Veterinary Science, Khanpara, Guwahati, Assam (AAU) 1969
35. Lakhimpur College of Veterinary and Animal Science, Lakhampur, Assam (AAU)*, 1987
36. Bihar Veterinary College, Patna (RAU) 1927
37. Faculty of Veterinary and Animal Hubandry, Kanke, Ranchi. (BAU) 1971
38. Dr. G.C. Negi College of Veterinary and Animal Sciences, Palampur (CCKHPKVV) 1986
39. College of Veterinary and Animal Sciences, Pantnagar, (GBPUAT) 1960
40. College of Veterinary and Animal Science, Junagharh (JAU)* 2008
41. College of Veterinary and Animal Science, Navasari*, Gujarat (NAU)* 2008
42. College of Veterinary Science & Animal Husbandry, Faizabad, UP (NDUAT) 1994
43. College of Veterinary Science & Animal Husbandry, Bhubaneswar, (OUAT) 1955
44. College of Veterinary and Animal Science, Meerut* (SBBPUAT) 2000
45. College of Veterinary Science & Animal Husbandry, S.K. Nagar, Dantiwara, Gujarat (SKAU) 1981

46. Faculty of Veterinary Science and Animal Husbandry, Sohama, (SKAUST-K) 1990
47. Faculty of Veterinary Science and Animal Husbandry, R S Pura (SKAUST-J) 1995

C. Veterinary College with Central agricultural University (CAU)

48. College of Veterinary Science & Animal Husbandry, Aizawl, Mizoram (CAU) 1993

D. Government Veterinary College-affiliated to General University

49. College of Veterinary and Animal Sciences, Agartala-affiliated to Tripura University (Central University) 2009
50. Rajiv Gandhi Institute of Veterinary Education and Research, Pondicherry (affiliated to Pondicherry University) 1994

E. Private Veterinary Colleges affiliated to SVUs

51. Apollo College of Veterinary Medicine, Jaipur[Δ] (RAJUVAS) 2003
52. M.G. Veterinary College, Bharatpur[Δ] (RAJUVAS) 2005
53. College of Veterinary and Animal Science, Sikar* (RAJUVAS) 2010
54. MJF Veterinary College of Chomu, Jaipur[Δ] (RAJUVAS) 2010
55. M.B Veterinary College of Dungarpur[ΔΔ] (RAJUVAS) 2011
56. B.S College of Veterinary Medicine and Research Institute, Mukand garh, Jhunjhunu* (RAJUVAS) 2010
57. S.G Veterinary College Sri Ganga Nagar* Affiliated to Pvt. University, Ganganagar 2010
58. Khalsa College of Veterinary Sciences, Amritsar* (GADVASU) 2010
59. SM College of Veterinary Science and Animal Research, Palidogra, Mathura* (DUVASU), 2009
60. International college of Veterinary Science and Animal Research Center, Rothak* (LUVAS), 2013

F. Deemed to be Universities of ICAR (DU) (dealing with post graduation education in Veterinary and Animal Sciences)

Indian Veterinary Research Institute (IVRI), Izatnagar, Bareilly UP Estt 1889 and DU 1983

National Dairy Research Institute (NDRI), Karnal, Haryana Estt.1923 and DU 1987

* not listed in First Schedule of IVC Act, 1984

Δ recognised upto 11.07.2011

ΔΔ recognised upto 08.12.2011

Note :

1 Kamdhenu University, Gandhi Nagar (Gujarat) created in 2009 is yet to establish a Veterinary College.

2 Some states are venturing to create Veterinary Colleges. New colleges that are in the process of establishment include, at Bilaspur-(CGKDVV), Rampuraphool, Bhatinda (GADVASU), Varanasi (BHU), Athini and Puttur (KVAFU).

□□□

Chapter-2

Resources at Command

This chapter deals with various types of resources needed for a viable veterinary institution viz. number and types of Institutions, infrastructural, human, livestock and financial resources required to manage education programs in veterinary and animal sciences. academic regulations & academic programs and the resultant beneficiaries - the students have been dealt with.

2.0 The success of any educational programs require available inputs in the form of adequately equipped institutions, sound programs that have social relevance & market acceptability, competence of organizational forces in qualitative and quantitative terms, basic ingredients- the students/trainees who are to be benefited from the programs/courses and availability financial back up to run the institutional programs on sustainable basis.

In context of veterinary education, the primary resources required to manage veterinary educational programs on sustainable basis are;

2.1 Educational institutions

2.2 Human resources

2.3 Students enrolment

2.4 Academic programs

2.5 Infrastructure including land, buildings, equipment, laboratories, class rooms, library, clinical and farm facilities and other support system

2.6 Livestock resources

2.7 Financial resources

The existing status of available resources is reflected in this chapter. However, resource management, primary issues and concerns with gap analysis as well as strategies to fill the gaps (where ever needed) are dealt in subsequent chapters.

2.1 Educational Institutions

Presently, there are in all 60 institutions (besides, 2 ICAR Institutes) in the country to cater to the needs of educational programs. Veterinary education is imparted mainly through State run institutions created under the broad umbrella of land grant system of education, while adhering to the principles delineated by the ICAR. Agricultural education inclusive of veterinary science is under the domain of State Governments. However, the ICAR being an apex coordinating organization of National Agricultural Research and Education system (NARES), has developed a Model Act for establishment of agricultural universities. The Model Act thus forms the basis of creation of state agricultural/ veterinary universities. Thus, all the agricultural universities legislated by the state assemblies are adhering to the broad provisions of the Model Act of ICAR. At present, 13 states have created veterinary and animal sciences universities (SVUs). Thirty two veterinary colleges are the constituents of these SVU while 15 colleges are constituent units of state agricultural universities (SAUs). One veterinary college is attached to the Central Agricultural University, one government college at Pondachery is affiliated to Pondicherry University and a college at Agartala is affiliated to Tripura University. In addition, there are 10 colleges established under private sector which have been affiliated to state veterinary universities (7 with RAJUVAS, one each with GADVASU, DUVASU and LUVAS).

Presently, some 34-35 colleges are enlisted in the First Schedule of the IVC Act, 1984. Enlistment of some colleges is in pipeline while some newly created colleges are yet to complete an academic cycle to become eligible to get recognition of their degree qualification. None of the college from private sector has been enlisted in the IVC schedule except Apollo at Jaipur and Mahatma Gandhi Vet. College, Bharatpur have been inducted in schedule-1 for a specified period under Hon'ble Supreme Court order. All colleges enlisted in the schedule are also offering master's and doctoral programs invariably in all the disciplines of veterinary and animal sciences. Four institutes namely Post Graduate Institute of Veterinary and Animal Sciences (PGIVAS), Akola, Post Graduate Institute of Veterinary Education & Research,

(PGIVER) Jaipur, Indian Veterinary Research Institutes (IVRI), Izatnagar and National Dairy Research Institute(NDRI), Karnal are exclusively offering PG education for the award of master's and doctorate degrees in veterinary and animal sciences. The NDRI do offer dairy technology degree course as well. PGIVAS, Akola is offering MVSc in 11 and PhD in 8 disciplines. Newly established PGIVER, at Jaipur presently is offering MVSc in LPM and Animal Nutrition. Ten post graduate departments are in the process of establishment namely Animal Nutrition, LPM, Veterinary Physiology & Biochemistry, Microbiology, Pathology, Parasitology, LPT, Livestock Extension Education, Animal Breeding & Genetics and Medicine

There are regional imbalances in distribution of veterinary and animal sciences universities and colleges across the country. All southern states have veterinary universities (TNVASU,KVAFU, SVVU KUVAS) in the respective states. Further, each of these states have reasonably good number of veterinary colleges (4,5,4,2 respectively). Recently established colleges are in growing stage while old colleges are sound in health and these possess the capacity and capabilities to impart quality education. On the contrary amongst the eastern states there is only one veterinary university at Kolkota in West Bengal and every state including WB has a single veterinary college except Assam having 2 colleges attached to SAU (one is still in infancy stage). Though, the Colleges of West Bengal and Patna are century old institutions credited with laudable past history but some way down the line these institutions now have lagged behind. Presently many other colleges in this part of the country are not able to sustain a very sound health status. In central part of India Maharashtra, MP and Chhattisgarh have veterinary universities with 6, 3 and 1 colleges respectively. North and Western part of the country have veterinary universities in Rajasthan, Haryana, Punjab and UP. Wide variability and uniqueness exists in this part of India with Rajasthan having 10 colleges including 7 from private sector and one post graduate institute-the PGIVER, Haryana and Punjab have one constituent and one Private Sector colleges in each, Himachal and J & K have colleges attached to SAUs. UP has a veterinary university with one college attached to it. There exist two more colleges in the state of UP which are constituent units of other SAUs of the state. One affiliated college from private sector was created at Mathura which has gone non- functional few years after its establishment. The Gujarat is the only state in the Country that had created Veterinary University, but all of the 4 existing

Veterinary colleges are continuing to be attached to the 4 SAUs of the state. The University is yet to create veterinary college even after its establishment in 2009. Amongst the existing veterinary universities two are mono-faculty (RAJUVAS & LUVAS), four having two DUVASU, NDVASU, CGKDVV, KVAFU) and rest are having all the 3 vital faculties (Veterinary, Dairy and Fishery).

India is proud to have some of the institutions matching global order. Quality of health services rendered to livestock, companion animals, birds, zoo and wild species is exceedingly good to satisfactory level in most of the established colleges. It is very much satisfying that most of the institutes have given priorities to update and modernize their teaching veterinary clinical complex (TVCC). The TVCC at Chennai, Mumbai, and Bangalore veterinary colleges are registering few hundred cases daily. Other amongst the potential clinical service units are at veterinary colleges at Bikaner, Ludhiana, Hisar, Mathura, Hyderabad, Mannuity, Jabalpur, Mhow, Orrisa etc. The most satisfying developments that have taken place during the last two decades have been construction and strengthening of TVCC that are adequately equipped with latest technologies. Newly created institutions at Shirwal, Udgir, Gyanwaram, Udaipur and some private colleges like Jaipur, Amritsar, Bharatpur, Sikar, Rohtak have established exceedingly good TVCC. The Veterinary College at Palmpur has created an excellent model of TVCC. Besides this, establishment of instructional livestock farm complex (ILFC) also remained a priority with veterinary Institutions.

Age old buildings of some colleges have outlived their utility. Structures are caving in and even the best of the facilities created during fifties and sixties have become unsuitable in present day context. Though, at stages these institutes got catch grants for repair, re-modulation, and modernization in form of grant in aid from ICAR or from state governments but such grants remained peanuts for gigantic structures. Many colleges are structurally weak and do not match to the desired standards to impart education. It is also true that new buildings that have been created during the last 25 years either at existing institutions or newly established institutions are by and large adhering to the prescribed standards of the VCI.

Location of some of the colleges has become permanent handicap. Since these have been located at remote areas away from habitation and animal population, routinely sufficient cases are not reported to effectively impart clinical training. Many colleges are located away from the city/ town and thus student, faculty and staff have to travel considerably to reach the destination. Some institutions have become permanently disabled for faulty selection of site of college/TVCC. A few institutes are compensating low turnout of clinical cases at the institutional TVCC, by according greater emphasis through ambulatory by extending health services at the door steps of the livestock owners. Students are also deputed for clinical services at the government multi facilities veterinary hospitals in the city.

Presently only 34-35 scheduled colleges are producing veterinary graduates. The total output from these colleges is;

- Graduates (BVSc&AH/BVSc 2,000
- Masters (MVSc/MSc) 750
- Doctorates (PhD) 150

The output from Veterinary Institutions is far less that the present day requirement. Such issues will be appropriately discussed in subsequent chapters.

List of Veterinary educational institutes is available at Annexure-1 of Chapter-1

2.2 Human Resource

Human resource is the key component of growth. The greatest asset of a nation is its human capital. The pathway for development is the availability of competent and qualified manpower, its effectiveness in ever changing needs, constant and regular flow of young talent so as to maintain a fair balance between highly experienced faculty, middle level functionaries and fresh talent to enable the system remaining productive at all times. Unfortunately such ideal situation is rarely visible even at the best of the institutes.

Universities/Institutes are the main hub for human resource development in any sector. Livestock sector is fast growing and transforming to shape as industry. The profile of the professional managing this sector is becoming more and more demanding as well as challenging. It is thus of a paramount importance that the teaching institutions should have optimum number of faculty possessing update knowledge, skills and competence.

The VCI as the supreme statutory authority has been entrusted with the responsibility to prescribe 'Minimum Standards of Veterinary Education-degree course (BVSc&AH), Regulations (MSVE). The manpower requirements to manage only undergraduate education for a batch of 60 students as per VCI norms are; 18 professors, 24 associate professor and 44 assistant professors. (These figures are inclusive of specialized cadres of hospital superintendent, farm managers etc). Further, extra manpower is required to manage PG teaching, research and transfer of technological practices. To manage teaching and research at all the veterinary institutes about, 7500 competent faculty is required as per the existing regulation. Against these, availability of faculty is only 3050. (< 50%)

There a very wide variability of human resource in terms of quality, quantity, cadre, discipline, region and even from college to college within the same university. Veterinary colleges at Assam, Tamil Nadu, Bangalore, Ludhiana, Hyderabad, Mannuty, Hisar, Triputi and at few more places may have fairly good number of faculty but even there exist imbalances in cadre strength and also on the basis of disciplines. Recruitment never remained a regular feature in most of the universities. Further, universities have failed to fill senior positions through lateral entry and there always remained paucity of available manpower in some of the emerging disciplines. Implementation of career advancement scheme (CAS) has tilted the pyramid with a heavy top and weak base. At certain institutes all available positions are manned only by professors. All are in position by virtue of CAS. Quantification in terms of number is difficult, but fairly old colleges at Ranchi, Shirwal, Udgir, Pakhot, Faizabad, Dantiwara etc. have number of available manpower much less than the desired standards. Manpower strength to lately established colleges at Rewa, Udaipur, Tripura, Sivamogga, Orathanadu, Tirunelveli, Korutla, Proddatur etc. are being geared up.

2.2.1 Induction Courses and competence enhancement programs for faculty/ scientist

The ICAR has structured induction courses primarily through the National Academy of Agricultural Research Management (NAARM), Hyderabad. It is highly satisfying that the new entrants in ICAR cadre through ARS have to undergo induction course which is highly useful for the freshers to get acquainted with the NARES system. During course of the training besides getting orientation with their job pursuits and expectation of the council from them they are exposed to governance mechanisms, financial management, socio economic scenario of rural developmental programs relating to agricultural sciences etc. Peer group of scientists from diversified spectrum are invited for interactive meetings with the participants. Some universities have also tied up with NAARM to manage Induction courses there. Certain universities have also created management academy. However, by and large, in Veterinary Universities, such practice is rarely seen.

The ICAR through their Education Division is organizing summer/ winter schools/short courses through the universities/ research institutes. ICAR in addition to bearing the entire cost of training also provide strengthening support to host universities. This year ICAR is organizing 44 winter/Summer schools of 21 days duration and 40 short courses of 10 days duration. Of these, 6 schools and 9 short courses relevant to the faculty of veterinary and animal sciences and allied sector shall be organized in SAUs/SVUs/Institutes.

Further, societies of every discipline are organizing annual symposiums/workshop etc. every year. It is a forum where scientist gets opportunity to present his/her work and a young scientist gets the pulse of national/international projections of scientific developments.

There are other opportunities available for potential faculty/ scientist to avail benefits of foreign travel to participate on international forums. Potential scientists get invitations to participate nationally and internationally on their own strength.

Over the times, the governments (union and states) and the universities have launched many beneficial schemes for faculty competence enhancement and up gradation of their qualifications, skills and competence. Some organizations have put in place incentive and rewards for outstanding faculty, introduced schemes of adjunct professor, emeritus scientist, national fellows sabbatical leaves etc.

In true analysis, the benefits of the aforesaid schemes are not percolating in veterinary and animal sciences to the extent it ought to have been. There are obvious reasons which make these benefits inaccessible to a veterinary teacher. Less availability of staff, resource crunch, lack or priorities of the institution and lack of transparency are creating hindrances in the system. It is equally true that scientist is rarely interested to avail benefits from national schemes but would like to grab every possible opportunity to avail international benefits. The overall scenario in translating national schemes on faculty competence improvements is not very encouraging owing to eruption of certain defects in the process of implementation of the scheme and by and large passive attitude of the faculty.

2.3 Students Enrolment

Entry level qualifications to BVSc&AH course is 10+2 with science (physics, chemistry), biology (botany, zoology) with compulsory English. To be eligible for admission one must have secured 50% marks at 10+2 or equivalent. Admissions to all colleges are made through entrance examination conducted in the respective states by an agency approved and authorized by the state government. Further, in order to reduce inbreeding, 15% seats are filled by the VCI through All India entrance test conducted by the VCI. The VCI allot candidate to the colleges that are enlisted in the First Schedule of the IVC Act, 1984. A batch of 60 students is admitted to each college. However, some colleges have been granted fewer admissions by the VCI based upon their available infrastructure and manpower. Reservation policy of the respective state government is followed by all the colleges.

Admissions to PG programs are made by the University while adhering to the ICAR norms. Admissions are made on the basis of merit or entrance test subject to the response and number of seats available. Twenty five per cent seats to each course are allotted by ICAR through All India entrance test for admissions and JRF conducted by it. At present ICAR award 475 JRF to the students of all faculties of agricultural sciences. The fellowship amount is Rs.12000 PM + Rs.5000 PA as contingency for veterinary students with a total no of JRF around 110 for Veterinary students. Likewise ICAR conduct All India competition examination (AICE-SRF) for award of SRF to pursue PhD degree course. Of the total 202 SRF, 48 are for the students pursuing PhD in veterinary and animal science subjects. In addition, 9 fellowships are available in dairy science and technology courses.

Admissions for master's courses to IVRI and NDRI are regulated by common entrance test and JRF conducted by ICAR for SAUs but for PhD program respective institute conduct entrance test and admit students on all India basis. All students perusing masters or doctoral programs at ICAR institutes get JRF/ SRF or institute fellowship. SRF amount for veterinary students is Rs.14000.00 for first two years and

Rs.15000.00 for the third year. In additions, Rs.10, 000.00 PA is given as contingency grant.

Total enrolments of students in veterinary and animal sciences at SAUs/ SVUs for UG programs are from 8,000 to 9,000 and for PG courses it is 2,000. Annual output in the country is less than 2000 graduates, around 750 masters and 150 doctorates in veterinary sciences.

2.4 Academic Regulations and Syllabus (Course contents)

Soon after the constitution of the VCI by the central government, it had prescribed 'Minimum Standards of Veterinary Education-Degree Course (BVSc&AH)', Regulations, 1993 (MSVE) as per the Section 22 of the Indian Veterinary Council Act (IVC),1984 These regulations primarily pertains to eligibility qualification, duration of degree course, criteria of selection, attendance requirements, migration rules, examination and evaluation, pass percentage etc. Further, it has prescribed course credit system, duration of semester and academic cycle. The courses of each discipline have been enlisted and detailed course contents specified. Regulations were also made with respect to infrastructure-buildings, laboratories, class rooms, equipment, manpower and qualification of the faculty.

A total duration of degree course is of 5 years inclusive of 6 calendar months internship on completion of entire course work. 17 departments were identified in regulation 1993 at a veterinary college. The total course load spread in 9 semesters was of 188 credits as per MSVE, regulations 1993. Broad distribution of credit load was; Basic veterinary courses-43, Pre-production/clinical courses-50, Animal husbandry courses-45 and Clinical and other courses-50. The distribution between theory and practical was 103:85

These Regulations were revised in 2008. Presently these regulations are in vogue in all the veterinary colleges in India which are awarding BVSc&AH degree. The following are some of the highlighting modifications brought in regulations 2008.

- Minimum numbers of departments have been reduced to 15 as against 17 earlier. Department of Physiology and Biochemistry as well as department of Clinical and preventive medicine have been merged
- Students failing in not more than 2 subjects is eligible for supplementary as against one subject in 1993 regulations

- Total credit load for degree requirement has been reduced from 188 to 174 credit hour.(Basic Vet.Subjects-38, Production subjects-38, Pre-clinical-41, Clinical-40 and TVCC-17 credits respectively)
- Department wise redistribution of credit load
- Certain courses have been merged/ amalgamated
- New courses on entrepreneur training, veterinarian in society introduced in 9th semester.
- Non- credit course on farm practice introduced in 3rd and 4th semester
- Compulsory non credit trainings programs introduced to inculcate spirit of self learning through virtual class room, distant learning, strengthening hands on training and learning to work in team in form of (i) Tracking program (ii) Study Circle (iii) Entrepreneur training.
- Minimum core skills for graduating students have been identified that form significant skill evaluation parameters during Internship
- Manpower and infrastructural needs have been re-tuned

In the process of implementations of MSVE, Regulations 2008 certain working constraints, drawback, and anomalies surfaced which are required to be addressed. Some of these are;

- Too many short courses. There are 22 two credit courses which is not an ideal situation.
- Lack of continuity of courses such as structural details (Anatomy) is taught at a later stage than teaching functional aspects (Physiology). Pathology courses are started before anatomy and physiology courses are completed. Many more such examples exist.
- Lot of time is wasted in managing two end semesters (internal) and one annual board examinations (external)
- Wide variations in clubbing of courses for annual board examinations. It is variable between single courses of 3-4 credits to 4-5 courses of 8-10 credits.
- Many of the instrument and equipment listed have gone obsolete. These are required be deleted and/or replaced with latest version.
- Human resource needs does not meet the workload norms of UGC, ICAR especially when it is assessed for UG teaching.

2.5 Infrastructure including Land, Buildings, Equipment, Laboratories, Class Rooms, Library, Clinical and Farm Facilities, and other Support System

More than anything else, the sustainability of a viable institution depends on the selection of location of a veterinary institution. It is required to be doubly ensured that institute should have easy access to the needed resources effectively. Physical creation of facilities would become futile if institute is not able to garner desired functional resources in terms of man, animal, material and accessibility. Teaching and training requires extensive exposure to clinical cases and thus location of the hospital should be in the vicinity of animal habitation There is left a very little scope of reversal towards betterment, if institution is created at a place which is not suited to house an institution that has to cater to the mandated function. Some live examples where location has been a limiting factors for effectively operation of veterinary college activities like Mohanpur campus at WB, Goaregoan at Mumbai, Navania at Udaipur, upper Joying at Lakhimpur, Kumargang, Faizabad etc. Many a time Institutions have been/ are being created on political as well as non-political considerations without caring for assessing its viability or suitability.

Availability of land is not a serious issue with most of the public run veterinary institutions but the suitability of land for housing needs of a veterinary institution has been a concern. Non- usable surplus land allotted to an institution becomes a liability rather than an asset.

Most of the institutions are housed in old buildings that have out lived their productive life or utility. Massive support is required for renovation/addition/alteration/re-modulation or even reconstruction. New buildings that have come up during last 2-3 decades are modern and as per the prescribed specifications. Care has been taken to keep a scope of expansion. The laboratories are spacious, airy and well illuminated.

During the last two successive five years plans, better support has percolated especially through 'Development Grants of ICAR' for strengthening laboratories, library, computerization and purchase of audio-visual aids. Signs for better facilities at most of the colleges are visible. However, still many colleges' lack minimum facilities for hands on training to graduating students. There are numerous reasons for deficient facilities in the laboratories. More than the non availability of financial resources, institute fail to accord priority to UG education. Further, instruments are discarded for want of minor repairs. Usually very meager budgetary provisions are available under repair and maintenance.

In the recent past, apart from regular funding for laboratory equipment under 'Development grants of the ICAR, many institutions/ departments got liberal support for purchase of sophisticated and costly equipment for research and PG education under RKVY and research grants from other funding agencies. Many institutions have been benefited in conducting research in cutting edge technologies and PG students are getting quality training. Those institutions that are having competent and qualified faculty/ scientist are making the better use of the facilities. However, it is equally true that many departments have pooled sophisticated equipments but these either have never been unpacked, or competent person is not available to handle these. It is true that at some colleges, many instruments are lying idle for want of improper support or proper place to house the equipment or for want of managing proper cable networking and or air conditioning etc. Many of the equipment have become outdated even without putting to proper use. Certain equipment have been procured but their utility is very limited or their operation is financially unmanageable. Installation of incinerator, digital X rays, auto-analyzer etc. only have their proper utility if sufficient cases/ sample are available so as the institute is able to recover part of the running cost from the clients.

2.5.1 Teaching Veterinary Clinical Complex (TVCC) is essentially a teaching, training cum service unit of a veterinary college. This is a coordinating unit of all clinical departments' viz. surgery, medicine, and gynecology. The para-clinical departments of pathology, microbiology, parasitology, physiology and biochemistry actively participate in clinical diagnostic work **(Reference may be made to chapter 11 to get further details on TVCC)**.

2.6 Livestock Resources

Before projecting general scenario of livestock status at teaching institutions, it would be in general interest to have a glimpse of national status of livestock and their contribution to rural dependant agricultural livestock system vis a vis national economy.

Livestock sector is one of the main pillars of India's agrarian economy, food and nutritional security and livelihood. Animal husbandry practices are more dependable avocation in farming sector than crop husbandry.

According to 19th Livestock census-2012 livestock population is close to 512.0 million besides about 729.2 million poultry. Large ruminants (cattle, buffalo, mithun and yak) accounts for 58.38% (299,9 million) of which cattle account for 190.9 million (151 million indigenous and 37.9 million cross bred) and buffaloes 108 million. Of the large population of cattle, only 23.1 million (11.6%) of indigenous cattle have been so far described and categorized into 44 different population including 37 distinct and registered breeds. Indigenous breeds are classified on the basis of their utility as milch breeds (Sahiwal, Red Sindhi,Gir and Rathi) dual purpose- milch and draft breeds (Tharparkar, Hariana, Kankrej, Deoni, Ongle, Dangi,Kerikatha etc.) and draft breeds (Halikar,Khilar,Nagori,Kangayam, Red kandhari etc.)

Small ruminant constitute around 37.15% (190.24. million-constituting 65.1 million sheep and 135.2 million goats) of the total livestock population. Pigs account for 10.3 million, camel for 0.40 million and equines 1.04 million.

India thus has the distinction of having largest population of livestock in the world (512.0 million). It accounts for 57.3% of the world buffalo population and 14.4% of the cattle population. Between the states MP has the highest cattle population of 21.9 million followed by West Bengal 19.1 million. Other states having more than 10 million cattle wealth are UP (18.8), Maharashtra (16.1); Rajasthan (12.12) and AP (11.22) Tamil Nadu (11.1) million respectively. Pure bred accounts for 53.79% in Gujarat, 45.74% in TN, 43.62 and 43.05 in Haryana of the total cattle population of the State. On the contrary Kerala has 89.52% and Punjab has 49.37% of cross bred cattle. Non-descript cattle population is over 69%. Jharkhand with 93%, MP 92%, WB 82%, Orissa 73%, Uttaranchal 78% are the major States having more than the national average of non descript cattle. Invariably NE states have high proportion of cross bred. Buffalo population is highest in UP 22.8 million followed by 13.3 million in AP. Total bovine population (cattle and buffalo) is highest in UP 42.69 million followed by MP 31.0 millions. Amongst the small ruminants sheep concentration is highest in AP 25.5 million followed by 11 millions in Rajasthan. While, goat dominating states are Rajasthan 21.5, WB 15.0 UP 14.8, Maharashtra 10.3 and Bihar 10.1 million respectively. Assam has maximum pig 2 millions followed by 1.3 million in UP and 0.8 million in WB. Equine dominating states are Rajasthan and J&K. 90% of the camels are found in Rajasthan. Small proportions of camel are found in the adjoining States of Rajasthan ie Haryana and Gujarat. Yak and Mithun are sporadic in NE states regions. Poultry dominating states are TN, AP, MS and WB.

N.B: State wise figures presented above are projection of census 2007. On the basis of the information available as of now, the total livestock population decreased from 529.7 million in 2007 to 512.1 in 2012. However, LS population registered increase in Gujarat (15.36), UP (14.01), Assam (10.77), Bihar (8.56), Meghalaya (7.41), Sikkim (7.96) and Chhattisgarh (4.34) percent respectively during this period. In spite of the fact that cattle and buffalo population has decreased in 2012 as against 2007 but it is noteworthy to state that number of animals in milk (cattle and buffalo) has increased from 77 million to 80.5. (an increase of 4.51%) The fall in population of large ruminants in this census is mainly due to decrease in male population while female population has marginally showed an increase.

Though, there is no great variability between equine population between the census of 2007 and 2012 (11.7 against 11.40) but total numbers of horses and mules have increased while that of donkey decreased considerably to the tune of 27.17%. Mithun has registered a growth rate of 12.7% Yak and camel have registered a negative growth rate to the tune of 7% and 22.5% respectively. Steep fall of almost one forth population of camel (from 0.517 to 0.400 million) is alarming. Poultry has registered growth rate of 12.39 % from the previous census. Pig population also showed decline to the tune of 10.37%.

The early figures available for census figures of 2012 are showing interesting trends. There is an increase of productive bovines while unproductive animals and males are being weeding out. The proportion of high producing cross bred have also showed an increase from 19.9 in 2007 to 26.3% in 2012.

Live stock sector is more dependable avocation. Average growth rate of this sector which during 1950-70 was just 1% jumped to 3.9 to 4.9 % during 1970-90. On the contrary there is a steep decline in growth rate of crop sector from 3.1 during 1950-60 to 1.9-2.2 during 1970-90. The share of livestock sector has grown to 30% from 14% during the last decade. LS sector now has a sustainable growth rate of 3.5%. Distribution of live stock is more egalitarian than land. It controls pro poor dependent economy where 75% of the livestock holders are landless or marginal farmers. It also plays an important role in gender and social equity.

As per report, India has generated a sum of Rs. 4590 billons (Rs. 4, 59,051 crore) accounting for 24.8% of the value of output from agriculture and allied sectors at current prices only through animal husbandry practices. The income generated from milk alone is estimated at Rs.2,28,809 crore which is higher than from paddy (ie.1,35,307), wheat (RS.1,03,266) or sugarcane (37,366). The progressive increase in the output of milk, meat, eggs, and fish has resulted into improvisation of per-capita consumption of these comodities thereby exhibiting a positive sign for ensuring nutritional security of masses.

Though India stands first in milk production globally (134 million tons during 2012-13) and there has been quantum increase of 6-7 times in the last 4 decades. Low average productivity of our livestock is a cause of concern. Research studies made during the last decade has demonstrated that many of the milch breeds have genetic potential to produce 2000 to 3000 liters of milk during lactation of 305 days. There is a need to exploit genetic potentials of these animals. Growth in livestock is rising at a steady pace. The growth is demand driven and increased production of animal produce has helped in raising the income of middle class rural households. Further, there has been greater awareness as well as increasing capacity towards consumption of quality animal origin proteins which is steadily changing food habits of people both in rural and urban populations, and thus with increased availability, utilization of food from animal origin is on the rise. However, in India there is a wide gap between the availability of quality food and the biological needs of man and animals.

2.6.1 Instructional Livestock Farm Complex (ILFC) Livestock at the institutional level is a must to provide the services of teaching in rearing of livestock species including poultry with the facilities of housing, feeding, breeding and management as per the MSVE regulations 2008. It should also facilitate the student to get acquainted with record keeping on all aspects of health status, production, nutritional managements etc. ILFC should also have storage facilities fo feed and fodder crops etc. It should essentially have (i) Animal production and management, (ii) avian production and management, (iii) Fish production management, and (IV) fodder production management units.

ILFC has been given a status of a teaching department with adequate infrastructure and manpower. The VCI has been very particular to have ILFC as per the prescribed standards. Many colleges do not have the facilities to the extent these are required. Universities/ Colleges do have farms and livestock research stations. Since these university farms are mandated to conduct research in focused areas and there is always a pressure on these farms to generate income, usually these units are not open for routine hands on training to the students. It is because of these reasons the institution of an independent ILFC was conceptualized. It is thus suggested to have an independent unit having all species of animal which could be used for training of students' right from handling, securing, casting, administration of drugs, feeding experimentation, surgical and gynecological intervention etc. Though, the ICAR is allocating funds of establishing and strengthening of instructional farms but such an independent arrangement of ILFC is occasionally seen at veterinary colleges. (Reference may be invited to see chapter 9 on ILFC).

2.7 Financial Resources

Veterinary educational institutions are state run organizations and thus primary support for sustainability of the universities/ colleges is provided by the state government. However, the philosophy behind creation of agricultural educational system per se is on the pattern of land grant system of education. The Central government also provides Grant-in-aid through ICAR for development and strengthening of educations in the institutions. It is also envisaged that these universities should generate internal resources. Although, major funds come from the states, but these allocations are barely meeting the establishment cost and universities are gasping for successful operation of its academic needs. The support coming from ICAR under 'Strengthening and Development Grant' to institutions though, meager but has been very critical. The level of funding for the SAUs/ SVUs which used to be to the tune of 5-10% of the total budget of the university has now risen to 25-35% during the last 2 plan periods. These figures are deceptive for some universities which have proliferated over the time and thus university allocations gets thinly distributed between colleges. Out campuses are always lagging behind than the colleges at the university headquarter. Basic amenities like hostels especially Girls hostels, Central Instrumentational facilities (CIF), computerization, and library etc. are usually inadequately available at the off campuses.

Since, the veterinary education is primarily a rural based education where students usually come from rural background and that too from the lower strata of the society, fee structure has to be kept low. Thus, to expect the universities to generate resources through fee is beyond imagination. The universities, thus should bank upon other measures to generate resources especially through farms, product sales, consultancy, professional services, running professional training programs and structuring self sustainable programs etc. Universities should also be pro-active in garnering private funding.

Presently there is very wide variability in total allocation of funds to various universities which ranges roughly between Rs. 30-Rs.150 crore. Though fund, allocation depends upon the age of the universities, number of campuses, numbers of programs, state government's priorities but it is a fact that those universities that are getting substantial and timely state support are better managed organizations. Further, institute health depends upon external funding through research grants. Even within the college, the departments having research projects are better managed. In the changing world order, it is expected that every scientist should generate funds from external funding projects so as to strengthen department/ college.

Finally, it cannot be denied that the profession has grown multifold over the times. However, under the ever changing scenario, the pressure is mounting on this sector. The brief account of available resources presented in this chapter clearly signals that there is deficient resources-may it be institutions, infrastructural needs, manpower compounded with financial crunch, are signaling drastic changes in our strategic approach for bringing wide spread developments. Unless the governments visualize the role of livestock sector, much beyond the agriculture system per se, owing to its much diversified additional responsibilities and allocate substantial funding make the professional contribution viable for expected growth on sustainable basis. It calls for an independent organizational system to effectively cater to the needs of this sector. The Union Government must device appropriate means to bring changes in the organizational structure in managing the affairs of livestock sector by providing complete operational independence.

❑❑❑

Chapter-3

Resource Management

Attempts have been made in this chapter to suggest certain measures to create viable veterinary educational institution as well as developing strategies for human resource development. Certain measures have also been suggested to attract students to this profession.

3.1 Educational Institutions

Presently the country is grossly deficient in institutions in its qualitative and quantitative term. Though there are 60 veterinary institutions (besides, IVRI & NDRI) but in fact only 35-40 colleges are producing graduates on regular basis. Further, numbers of colleges offering PG programs are far more less. In true sense, colleges offering M.V.Sc and Ph.D with optimum infrastructural facilities inclusive of competent and qualified PG faculty covering all disciplines or veterinary and animal sciences sector may not be more than 25 (including IVRI and NDRI). The total out- turn of graduates and post graduates is insufficient to meet the national/ regional/ local demands. Under the global umbrella, Indian educational institutions generally are of no match to the advanced countries for want of sufficient numbers of competent and qualified faculty, especially in cutting edge technologies, and sub-optimal infrastrture. The VCI has laid down MSVE, Regulations. These are mandatory to be followed by all the colleges. Needless to mention that even the best of the institutions, are not able to fulfill these regulations (especially manpower and infrastructure) in its true perceptive.

Our approach should be to double the human capital by 2025. It is a herculean task and requires a cohesive approach between centre and states and it calls for a very meticulous planning and targeted roadmap. Some steps need to be initiated immediately to overcome the acute crisis. There is a need to identify potential colleges and based upon the available infrastructure, manpower and other resource, intake capacity for UG course may be raised from 60 to 90-120. In doing so the university/state government/ICAR should provide substantial support for capacity enhancement. Simultaneously it would be prudent and purposeful to make an in-depth analysis on need assessment and manpower planning. In planning processes, national, regional and sectoral priorities are to be kept in mind. Corrective steps may be taken to reduce regional imbalances. High priority states (livestock dominant areas) should be accorded priority in addressing these issues. The following measures would prove beneficial in building human capital of the desired status.

3.1.1 Every state of the country should have a functional veterinary university mandated to cover diversified spectrum of education and training in veterinary, animal sciences and allied sectors. No veterinary college/institution from this sector should be allowed to function outside the ambit of veterinary university of the state. (All veterinary colleges of Gujarat and two colleges of UP should be placed under the fold of veterinary universities of the respective state)

3.1.2 Central Veterinary Universities/Institutes should be created on regional/zonal basis on the pattern of AIIMS.

3.1.3 There is a need to create additional 50-60 more veterinary colleges in next one decade. In this regard joint efforts are called on massive scale from the centre, state governments, the VCI, the ICAR and private sector organizations.

3.1.4 Revival of non-performing or underperforming colleges should be taken on two fronts. On one side these colleges should be liberally supported to strengthen infrastructural needs and recruit manpower to fulfill the basic needs while on the other side the regulatory system may permit certain relaxation (without compromising on quality output) and allow colleges to build strength and capabilities in a specified time frame.

3.1.5 Developing and strengthening of 'Public Private Partnership' is required to be geared up. Government may prepare sound models for developing institutions under PPP mode.

3.1.6 It should also be explored to rope in potential players in private sector or the existing institutions may develop some vital activities under PPP mode. Institutions may venture to make ultra modern clinical services (multi specialty hospitals) through the participation of private sector. Institutional farms can also be modernized under PPP mode. There is a dire need for changing conceptual approach by re- defining mechanisms for developing lasting relationship with private sector. The universities are required to participate in developing private sector organizations by providing expertise and assisting them in managing their technical affairs.

3.2 Human Resource Development

3.2.1 Veterinary education is undergoing transformation. Under the changing scenario, veterinary graduates need orientation toward professional competence, self reliance and self confidence to enable them to be attractive towards cooperate sector or take up self employment, rather than dependent on public sector employment only. This is an audacious task that require meticulous planning along with strategic shift in approach. In this context a strong human resource programs have to be placed at the centre stage. Human resource development (HRD) is thus the greatest challenge being encountered by veterinary professional manage mental system. The institutions responsible to generate human resource, are in itself grossly deficient in qualified and competent faculty, besides, being improperly equipped with modern infrastructure and other pre-requisites. The country is deficient in number of institutions and faculty and thus their resultant output is low. Shortfalls in terms of availability of professional *vis a vis* their need is widening year after year.

It has been documented time and again by expert committees, academic managers and regulators that there exists a wide gap between demand and supply of human resource. Acute deficiency of manpower has been reflected in the document prepared by the Working Group on Animal Husbandry and Dairying in its report for 12th Five Year plan (2012-17) to the Planning Commission, GOI, on the human resource requirement and the availability of manpower in veterinary and animal husbandry sector. Merely **exhibiting concerns on the shortage of human capital by the central and or state regulatory organizations are of little value if concrete road maps in**

strengthening and creation of newer institutions to cover up the short falls are not put in place concurrently.

During the recent past, the central government, department of animal husbandry, dairying and fisheries (DAHDF) and the VCI conducted several national meets and constituted high powered expert committees, but follow up that ought to have shown tangible effects, are hardly visible. Further, the type of coordination between different regulatory authorities has not reached to the extent it is desired.

The attention of the authorities is drawn toward the general concern over the availability of human capital in higher education by Dr. Manmohan Singh, former Prime Minister on the news report in Times of India dated 29.12.2013 entitled **"UGC must look into faculty crunch: PM"**

Some of the extracts of his advice that has relevance to veterinary educational system are;"Singh asked the regulator to play the role of national 'think tank' and organize a professional and purposeful discourse about issues that have a close bearing on the sound management of higher education system".

Singh said that shortage of faculty in higher educational institutes is a serious problem that is likely to become more acute with the expansion. "Singh called for strengthening university-industry inter-phase to give boost to research and development. Greater support from industry will not only lead to better research outcome but also enable industry to utilize for meaningful practical application." **It would be prudent if the national regulatory authorities of this sector act on the advice of the former PM and draw road maps for speedy development. Corrections wherever needed must be applied to make the system more vibrant, productive, purposeful and shall be able to swiftly address to ever changing needs for the societal up-liftment.**

3.2.2 National challenges

To harness the animal husbandry sector for further growth and contribution to rural livelihood, human resource development is a vital factor, particularly at this junction of time when the country is in the midst of an agrarian crisis. About 20.6 million workers are involved in farming of animals. India with only 2.29% of the land area of the world, is maintaining about 10.71% of the global livestock population.

India has 10,317 veterinary hospitals/polyclinics, 22,713 veterinary dispensaries, 22,794 veterinary aid centers and 77,765 artificial insemination centers offering veterinary services to millions of farmers and livestock owners. The human resource requirement and availability in respect of veterinary and animal science to meet the need for research, academic and development has been worked out by the Institute of applied manpower research (IAMR) and NAARM (ICAR institute) in the year 2010. Very recently in 2011, the Working Group on Animal Husbandry and Dairying has also submitted its report for 12th Five Year plan (2012-17) to the Planning Commission, Government of India on the human resource requirement and the availability of manpower in veterinary and animal husbandry sector.

In the report of Working Group on A.H. & Dairying, 2011, it has been clearly indicated that against the requirement of 67,000 veterinarians, only 34,500 are available. Similarly, against the requirement of 7500 veterinary and animal science specialists for teaching and research, only 3050 are available. The other sectors where veterinarians are expected to play important role are; wildlife, bio-security and public health, veterinary extension, forestry, Insurance and industries like dairy, meat, poultry, pharmaceutical, animal feed industries, all India civil services and defense.

To bridge the wide gap between the currently available faculty strength in the veterinary colleges/institutes including deemed universities offering undergraduate and postgraduate programs and the available manpower, there is a need to have at least 4,450 more teaching veterinarians in addition to attrition and retirement rate of 3%. In order to support the increasing need, an aggressive approach is required. Thus, it is essential to strengthen the faculty position in existing colleges to produce the required manpower to manage both UG and PG teaching and research responsibilities.

Further, more and more teaching and training institutes are required to be created. However, the entire burden cannot be sustained by the public sector organizations alone and thus involvement of private sector is of paramount importance. Government should be serious in adopting a pro-active approach in developing 'Public Private Partnerships' (PPP). There is a need to energize private partners so that their participation would complement the public sector. Shri Ratan Tata recently made a welcome announcement that he wish to establish a veterinary poly-clinic and research center of global order at Mumbai.

Governments must tap some big giants to create such institutions in the country. The possibilities may be explored to have such units under PPP mode. In such a situation where expansion is needed at a faster pace, the quality assurance of education should be ensured at all levels.

Both the central and states governments should provide substantial funding to effectively manage human capital, in creating veterinary hospitals and associated units as per the realistic needs of present and future. Further, funds should be made available to improve infrastructure of the existing establishments as per the regulatory norms. Many hospitals particularly located in remote and difficult areas are not adequately equipped and lack basic amenities. The universities/institutes should be charged with the responsibilities to generate internal resources to the tune of 10-15% of the annual budget in order to cope up in meeting contingent demands.

3.2.3 Strategies to manage human resource for service sector

Highly skilled and competent professionals are of paramount significance in every sphere, but to manage educational institutions including research and technological driven areas, specialized cadre strength with higher qualifications (post-graduation-preferably PhD) is pre-requisite, while for rendering field services (service sector), major work force is constituted by veterinary graduates. Time of course demands more and higher qualified individuals to take care of health and management services at veterinary hospitals, animal farms, A.I centers and other allied field service units with basic qualification of graduation. Besides, there is need for specialized cadre to manage expertise services like poly clinics, diagnostic centers, biological product divisions, research units/farms, policy planning and managers etc. For such like focused professional activities, the qualifications have already been laid down/need to be delineated as per the needs of assigned responsibilities.

3.2.4 HR for Academic institutions

Academic institutions including scientific organizations and the personals managing these are the builders of the national wealth consisting of professional, material building and livestock production thereby raising socio-economic status of livestock owners. It is of utmost importance that the teaching and research institutes should be of high order with competent and qualified manpower for ensuring delivering quality education and research. Further, since research is the mandatory requirement as partial fulfillment of PG degrees, the institution/department offering PG programs should have a sound research base. Particularly faculty compitence & strength, infrastructure, adequate funding and condusive environment.

The policies and programs in the organization should be conducive for recruitment and retention of faculty. Merely inducting manpower without ensuring for quality would amount to compromising with the standards. Such practice would breed mediocrity in the system. There is thus a need for a very cautious approach in man power planning and phasing out institutional developmental programs as per the need and availability of resources. A proper balance has to be kept between demand and supply. Mushrooming of institutions with sub-optimal facilities or resources or compromising with the quality of human resource would be counterproductive. For ensuring human resource quality, faculty competence programs, exposure of working in centers of higher learning at national and international level, provision of sabbatical leave, visiting professorship and developing linkages etc. need to be put in place.

3.3 Students Enrolment

It cannot be denied that veterinary profession is still not a natural choice for the biological group of students coming after 10+2 board examination. In fact many pass out especially from urban areas are unaware of this profession as a potential alternate choice to pursue education in this field. And those who have knowledge about it mostly coming from rural set up are mostly reluctant to join veterinary course. Beside these, some of the other negative factors are;

3.3.1 There is overall shift of preferences for biology group of students. The trend to opt for biological science has receded over the years. Students are keen to shift to newer branches implied with global transformation and ICT revolutions. Technological driven, courses, namely social and environment sciences, international trade, international economics and business management, space sciences, radiation biology etc are the courses that have flooded the market. Most of these programs are controlled by private systems who have adopted aggressive approach in marketing these programs being run globally. These programs are of shorter durations and are linked with attractive placements. Further, there is a great amount of flexibility in eligibility cretaria, duration and other conditions.

3.3.2 It is equally true that medical field being the primary choice for biology group students, thus with the increase in number of colleges both in medical and dental colleges, these students consider these disciplines a better opportunity to pursue education in medicine or dental. It is merely the left out from these opt for veterinary course. These students are relatively of lower strata from amongst the10+2 passed out.Numbers of seats available in all veterinary college are much below in meeting national demands.

3.3.3 Approach to attract talent

3.3.3.1 Dr. M.S. Swaminathan committee report on 'Education for Agriculture: Bridge to a century of hope on the farm front' (1997) made a recommendation on exploring feasibility of introducing agricultural education at 10+2 level or at pre-high school level.

3.3.4.2 Veterinary colleges should organize awareness courses in schools. Career guidance centers of the universities/ institutes should undertake awareness amongst the students and their parents on importance of farm education.

3.3.3.2 Veterinary colleges should organize some function, elocution contest relevant to livestock, exhibitions, skill competence, animal welfare camps for school children etc.

3.3.3.3 Liberal National scholarships may be offered to attract students to join veterinary education.

N.B The author has relied upon the policy document of NAVS (I) on 'Human Resource Development in Veterinary Education' and (II) Trasforming Veterinary and Animal Science Education for Reshaping India's Economy by M.P. Yadav and J.S. Bhatia in 11th Agricultural Science Congress - NAAS Publication 2014.

❑❑❑

Chapter-4

Reforms in Veterinary Education (Academic Programs)

This chapter deals with suggestive reforms in veterinary educational programs especially by exploring the possibilities of introducing diversification in the degree program.

4.1 Introduction

Time demands changes which are inevitable. Through, it is difficult to affect the changes and simultaneously translate these in ever changing environment. However, it is not impossible, provided one has the 'will', determination and possesses positive frame of mind to do so. Education is key component for growth and a pre-requisite tool for bringing transformation. Educationist is primarily a learner. Apart from his being abreast with in-depth and latest knowledge, one must possess the capacity and capability to swiftly adjust to the changing environment and shall have the capacity to translate it into proper format for action. Dissemination of knowledge for its effective delivery for appropriate utilization is pre-requisite quality of an educator. Knowledge is expanding very fast and thus, to effectively assimilate and disseminate the knowledge, require up scaling/ modification of educational programs as and when the time demands. Veterinary educational system, like any educational programs, need frequent up gradation/modifications suiting to the relevance to time, region, AH practices and consumers demand.

4.2 Veterinary academic programs thus must be made relevant to meet market demands. The following issues are critical in revamping the system;

- Updating academic regulations and curricula in tune to the market demands

- Flexibility
- Multi-disciplinary and integrated approach
- Greater exposure/attachment to the relevant industrial houses, on farms training, co-operative societies, livestock marketing boards etc.
- Incorporating value addition and skill development courses/ programs.
- Re-introducing 'Earn while you learn' or practical on farm/ hospitals training with inbuilt incentives.

It is not that, needed changes have not been addressed and adjusted in the curriculum from time to time but to match the ever expanding role and responsibilities of a veterinarian and to equip him with the needed knowledge, skills and tools, there is a need for radical changes in veterinary educational program. Time has come to evaluate the relevance of the degree awarded in present day context. Rather than making cosmetic changes here and there in the course contents, the total system including eligibility criteria, duration, nomenclature of the degree courses and their contents, introducing flexibility in the program, delivery system, means and methodologies to equipping professional knowledge and skills etc. have to be taken into consideration simultaneously. It is equally important that some vital components from earlier educational systems that had been weeded or lost their identity over the times during restructuring degree courses are required to be reviewed. When one looks back, deletion of some components may have proved costly. We should not shy away in reverting back to those essential elements that still are needed to make sound base for the knowledge and training. At stages, few of the traditional wisdoms still have relevance in present day context. These are required to be seen and accommodated under scientific umbrella.

Exercise to revamp veterinary education system needs voluminous efforts with wider participation that are required to be seen from multi-dimensional angles. The existing system does have some provisions for consultations between various functionaries and stake holders but if the institutions are expected to abruptly adapt to the proposed change without allowing them to create pre-requisites resources to match the needs to translate new format effectively than the resultant outcome are bound to be below par. Further, to test the practical feasibility of revised model, feedback mechanisms are required to be built in the system. The authorities should be open for remedying the serious setbacks, if any, that might erupte in translating changes in operation of the program. Strict enforcement of the regulations of course are the responsibilities of regulatory authorities but rigid posture some time proves counterproductive. The system must have inbuilt mechanisms for mid-course corrections.

The Regulations framed under VCI provide every minor detail in terms of syllabus, course details, academic regulations, infrastructure and manpower needs etc. The program has been made almost water jacketed and the course load is so heavy that it becomes difficult for the institution to accommodate additional courses to the students. In fact a stereotype program is offered throughout the country in spite the fact that wide variability exists between the colleges even within the university with respect to the level of available competence, infrastructure and other facilities colleges. Students undergoing education from PG departments are bound to get a better exposure than the ones who are pursuing education at undergraduate college. It is also true that the academic bodies of the universities (academic council, board of studies, faculties and committee of courses) are having very little role in planning and execution of BVSc&AH degree program since MSVE, Regulations are guiding force which in practice is followed as such.

The VCI through its Regulations should restrict itself in defining academic regulations in term of eligibility criteria, duration of degree program, course credit distribution courses (core courses) and leaving at least 30% of the courses for the university to decide depending upon regional priorities, employment opportunities and the strength of the university. The regulations should provide credit hours, objectives and practical skill needed for each course. The existing VCI regulations have already identified minimum core skills needed for a graduate on the basis of which the interns are evaluated for successful completion of BVSc&AH degree. These skills can be further modified and enlarged to make training more purposeful. The procedure for evaluation can be made more rigorous to ensure that there is no scope for the graduating student to escape from acquiring pre-requisite knowledge and skills. However, it should be left to the university to detail out the courses contents of the prescribed courses, develop guidelines and their semester wise placement during the degree program while adhering to the laid down provisions of VCI regulations. University should also be given more flexibility as well as academic autonomy so that it gets opportunity to show its strength/uniqueness in identified area.

The primary responsibility of a veterinarian is animal health care and management of animals. This aspect should not be lost sight while making structural changes to the basic degree course(s). The existing program is already over loaded. A proper balance is required to be struck while affecting vital transformations. The total situation has to be assessed from multiple angles. One of the following broad approaches (or any other alternative) could be critically examined for adoption to bring desired changes.

- Should there be modifications in the existing course curriculum and academic regulations to the degree program in vogue with some addition and deletion of courses / contents as has been the practice in the past or an elaborate exercise be made for making drastic changes ?

OR

- Making room for diversification within the same degree course after imparting core competence of knowledge and skills for initial period of 3 years or so.

OR

- Should there be separate degree courses in broad disciplines of veterinary and animal husbandry sector?

OR

- Would it be feasible to integrate courses from different degree programs /faculties or even outside the university jurisdiction?

OR

- Should it be possible to introduce dual degree programs with multiple entry and exists?

A very cautious approach is required while introducing new degree course(s). Its market feasibility is required to be assessed on long term perspective. We have had unpleasant experience of starting B.Sc in Animal Sciences degree course which did not yield desired result and the program had to be dropped. Pulse of the industry and other end users is required to be assessed before starting new programs. Industries are opening to induct graduates but still veterinary graduates are not fully tuned to work in industrial set up. Participation of Industries in academic planning and execution of programs should be strengthened.

There is thus a dire need to restructure our degree program so that we are able to produce veterinarians who could be equipped to cater to the responsibilities in different professional arenas including industries, entrepreneur-ship etc.

4.3 In this direction a model has been presented for possible restructuring veterinary degree course. This may be modified/ improvised with wider consultation

- Degree program should be restructured by incorporating greater flexibility and wide variability. Instead of a single degree course in vogue, program should have inbuilt mechanisms to impart basic knowledge and skills in veterinary and animal science, besidedes allowing graduates to be equipped in certain identified areas for acquisition of specific skills (**professional focus**). At the initial stage, three tracts are proposed to be identified (which can be further expanded in due course of time) such as (i) Animal health (ii) Livestock production sciences (iii) Livestock product processing.(technology driven).

  The degree course is thus divided in three phases viz.

  a. **Compulsory core courses** for 3 years

  b. One year program on **professional focus** (60% courses from main area-professional focus and 40% from rest two areas.

  c. Last year should be earmarked for adjusting courses on **area of application** (one semester) internship or skill empowerment (based upon professional focus and its application (one semester).

Area of application could be

Health group; Pet (companion) animals, large animals, equines, wild and zoo animals, orthopedic, diagnostics, public health & zoonotic diseases, pharmaceuticals, indigenous medicine etc.

Production group; Species specific specialization, nutrition, breeding & genetics, production physiology, feeding technologies, LS economics and marketing, business management and social sciences.

LS Product technology; meat technology, milk technology, quality control, wool, fur and fiber technologies, leather, skin, hide, dung and urine technologies.

The VCI should identify course objective and outline, while it should be left to the universities to develop course contents. Further, universities should be free to add 25-30% courses especially in areas of professional focus and in area of application based upon its strength.

Special grants may be given for each college to develop facilities and expertise in identified areas of professional focus and area of application. Changes in nomenclature of the degree may appropriately be considered.

4.4 Examinations and Evaluation Reforms

Presently the examination system as per the MSVE, Regulations, 2008 needs a thorough insight. To conduct two end semester internal examinations (one in each semester) of individual courses from a department and an annual composite paper (amalgamated course (s) of each semester from a department) is not only time consuming process but does not serve any useful purpose of repeating examination one after the other (both of theory and practical) especially in second semester. The End semester examinations and annual external examinations are managed within a gap of a week to 10 days between the two, serve no useful purpose but merely a waste of time. In a situation when there is a single course in first semester with none in second semester, one has to take internal end semester in first semester and the external examination for the same is repeated at the end of second semester ie the student has to appear for external examination after a gap of 5 months of the course he has completed in first semester. In one academic year almost 3 months are utilized for examinations which is a colossal waste of time.

A committee is required to be constituted to suggest reforms for examination and evaluation system. Academic regulations pertaining to examinations are also required to be seen a fresh.

4.5 PG Education

PG education presently is regulated through ICAR-SAU/SVU system. The VCI had made a mammoth exercise to draft PG regulations and widely circulated for suggestions and comments more than a decade back. However, this exercise has lost its momentum and now there is a complete silence over this issue by the VCI. It will be in professional interest if there is proper synchronization of higher education (UG and PG) in totality. Revamping of degree course will add value only if it is linked with PG programs as well.

As of now veterinary universities are moving in a narrow spectrum by restricting itself maximally to dairy technology and fishery sciences, besides imparting veterinary and animal science education. These Universities have to UNIVERALISE EDUCATION AND TRAINING IN LIVESTOCK SECTOR WHILE ENCOMPASSING ON THE DIVERSIFIED BOUNDRIES OF THIS SECTOR. Programs should be technology driven, tuned to fulfill Industrial needs, besides the graduates to be thoroughly equipped with latest and innovative skills. Every university should develop unique character through which it must have a national and global recognition with a stamp of excellence. Universities of course are duty bond to keep their programs at the backdrop of the national regulatory standards on education while introducing any educational programs.

PS. Some reflections on PG education are dealt in the next chapter.

❑❑❑

Chapter-5

Post Graduate Education in Veterinary & Animal Sciences (Academic-degree programs, PG diploma & Continuing Veterinary Education)

Attempt has been made in this chapter towards developing some pre-requisite standards for running PG academic degree courses and need for structuring of continuing veterinary education (CVE) especially for service sector.

5.1 Status of PG Education (M.V.Sc and Ph.D)

Post Graduate education presently is regulated through ICAR-SAU/SVU system. The VCI had made a mammoth exercise to draft PG regulations and widely circulated it for suggestions and comments more than a decade back. However, this exercise has lost its momentum and now there is a complete silence over this issue by the VCI. It will be in professional interest if there is proper synchronization of veterinary education (UG & PG) in totality and revamping of degree course (BVSc&AH) will add value only if it is linked with PG programs.

PG education is offered in 30-35 veterinary colleges in the country, besides, two ICAR institutes (IVRI & NDRI). In addition there are two PG institutes, one Post Graduate Institute of Veterinary and Animal Science (PGIVAS) at Akola, (MAFSU) MS established in the year 1970 and the other recently established Post Graduate Institute of Veterinary Education and Research (PGIVER) at Jaipur(RAJUVAS) established in 2012. The PG program is governed through integrated participation of the ICAR and the state agricultural/veterinary universities where MVSc and Ph.D programs are offered in 17-23 disciplines at different institutions. The ICAR has formulated academic regulations, uniformly applicable for all disciplines and drawn course credit as well as syllabus of 18 disciplines of veterinary and animal sciences through the participation of Broad Subject Matter Area Committees (BSMA). The recommendations of BSMA has been accepted by the accreditation board of ICAR and implemented by most of the universities. The ICAR has built in financial support to the universities who have implemented BSMA recommendations.

The IVRI and the NDRI are the ICAR institutes having 'Deemed to be University' status granted by the UGC. By virtue of these, they have their own academic regulations. The IVRI offers M.V.Sc and Ph.D in 23 major disciplines. Beside IVRI offers National Diploma course for field veterinarians in 09 areas and short term training courses for the benefit and enhancement of knowledge of veterinarians and other research personals working at field level in livestock farms, disease investigation/diagnostic laboratories and veterinary colleges/ laboratories. The NDRI offers M. Sc Dairying and Ph.D in 10 disciplines of dairy/animal sciences/technology that have a relevance to veterinary qualification.

Until the recent past, there were no standard norms prescribed for PG education and thus there remained a great variability with respect to infrastructure, manpower and other facilities with university to university and college to college. Now academic regulations and course contents are by and large uniform as per ICAR norms. Though, some of the colleges are running masters and/or doctoral programs with adequate laboratory and optimum infrastructural facilities, while at number of other institutions, PG programs are offered with hardly few teachers that too are of junior cadres with limited facilities. It is because of these handicaps, in such institutions, quality output is below par. Recently the education division of ICAR through its accreditation section has constituted a committee to work out the 'Minimum Standards for higher education in veterinary and animal sciences'. Reference in this chapter has been made to some of the recommendations of ICAR committee.

PG education is a research based educational programs and thus there is a need for strategic shift in the approach while transforming higher educational system. Research and education are complimentary to each other. Thus higher education has been planned in a way that PG student is exposed to knowledge and skill acquisition on one side and conduct meaningful research under the guidance of expert faculty on the other. PG degree programs thus have fairly a good blend of teaching and research programs. There is relatively greater emphasis on course work in master degree program while for PhD, emphasis is shifted towards higher research credits load over course work. It is required to be ensured that PG student should be extensively exposed to quality hands on training. He should be able to make practical application of knowledge and skills acquired during training. Further, through understanding of instrumentation should be considered mandatory. At M.V.Sc. level the scope of the research should be limited up to understanding and identify the problem and be able to investigate and analyze with appropriate and approved methodologies. However, at Ph.D level much emphasis is required for research work and student should be held more accountable for detail exploration of the subject chosen. A web based *POSTGRADUATE RESEARCHPEDIA* should be created and all research work conducted under NARES system should be uploaded to avoid duplicity and maintain transparency and accountability.

On the pattern of the practice that is followed in medical sciences the regulators should explore the feasibility of **Residency Services** in areas of poly-clinics, Dairy processing plants, Meat Processing enterprises, Wool industry, Food safety laboratories, Animal Feed manufacturing factories, various livestock farms including stud and poultry farms, Diagnostic laboratories, Research & Development houses of Industries, Reputed NGO's and other related enterprises of veterinary and Animal husbandry. The pragmatic solution for such arrangement is that if the university should make structural arrangements for residency with government or corporate or any voluntary organizations. There should be an inbuilt arrangement of stipend/ assistantship etc. Such arrangements would enhance confidence building besides making him accountable.

In a dynamic educational system, courses are updated/revised every 5-7 years. Normally in the process of re-organization of PG education in veterinary and animal sciences, the course contents are modified/updated. This exercise gives leverage to modify the academic regulations as per the needs. However, no explicit guiding principles have been developed or laid down for research pursuits except for allocating credits and manner of conduct of synopsis preparation, theses seminar/evaluation etc.

PG department thus must have a sound research base. Besides, having optimum facilities and manpower as per the prescribed norms, the department must be actively involved in research. Every PG department must have developed research priorities in specified area for the next 10 years. These priority areas should have approval of academic/research advisory council. There is need to have active research operational in the form of projects (internal/external aided) in these priority areas. Students are expected to perform theses research well within priority research areas. Further, there should be continuity of student research problem one after the other. To encourage students for working in the project, positions of graduate assistance-ship/ fellowship should be made available. Student research should primarily have broad application to serve towards industry requirement or farmer based integrations.

ICAR has done a recent exercise to draw 'Minimum Standards of Higher Agricultural Education' (MSHAE) for all the 12 faculties of Agricultural Sciences. A committee was constituted to lay down the minimum standards for veterinary education. This committee was expected to work in different dimensions than the other faculties owing to the fact the Veterinary Council of India (VCI) has the statutory authority to prescribe the Minimum Standards of Veterinary Education-degree course (BVSc&AH), Regulation (MSVE). This committee while honoring the MSVE, Regulations of the VCI for degree course, has worked out to recommend 'Minimum Standards for PG education in veterinary and animal sciences' over and above MSVE, regulations, 2008 of the VCI. The report of the committee is in process of implementation by the accreditation section of Education Division of ICAR. This committee has made recommendations with respect to infrastructural requirement, human capital, livestock resource and other common facilities like centralized instrumentation facilities, library, animal farms and adequate financial backup etc. Readers are requested to visit MSHAE for veterinary and animal sciences of ICAR in this connection.

5.1.1 Optimum requirements for PG education

PG departments should have certain basic pre-requisite infrastructural needs, besides competent and qualified PG faculty. There should be a separate PG cum research laboratory, seminar hall and certain essential centralized facilities like experiment animal house, Central library, Central instrumentation facilities (CIF), PG hostels etc. CIF should have provisions of all types of Microscopes (high end research, binocular, UV, dark field, inverted, phase contrast, stereo zoom etc) and Histo-Pathology units (cryostats, freezing microtome), analytical equipment (colorimeters, spectrophotometers, AAS, HPLC, real time PCR, flame photometers, Elisa reader etc) centrifuges (refrigerated, ultra and high speed), freezing unit, lyophilizer and cooling units, weighing balances, water distillation, Millipore distillation unit and deionizers, ovens and Incubators (CO_2, BOD, digital shaking water bath) etc. There should be separate allocation of funds for PG teaching and research.

5.2 Continuing Veterinary Education- PG Diploma courses especially for service sector

There is an organized network of universities and colleges through which degree programs in higher education-academic stream operates in the country. The status of Institutions and institutional degree programs has been dealt in earlier chapters. However, equally important obligation of the Governments, regulatory authorities and universities is to structure programs for enhancing/updating the competence of professionals engaged in service sector. There are thus compelling reasons to urgently look at **'Continuing Veterinary Education' (CVE).**

CVE can be defined as the educative process enabled by accredited institutions in which professionally qualified veterinarian continue formally or informally be educated through an instructive process to improve his/ her professional competence.

This process can be achieved by a periodic on-campus, distance or remote, or a mixed on-campus and off-campus programs of study. These have to be distinguished from higher education that leads to a Diploma, Master's or Doctorate degrees, which usually are on-campus full time programs. However, in some CVE programs, credits earned by these studies can lead to a recognized specialization or a post graduate degree/Diploma. In some cases, a certain amount of education is continuously required to be credited to a specialized discipline or professional specialty.

The CVE in Indian context has relevance as continuous efforts required on large scale to optimize productivity and enhance product quality. Professional competence enhancement of massive work force involved in delivery of services in live stock sector is a real challenge. Better and better professional services in this sector are all the more demanding since food crop production is almost touching plateau and to target 4 plus economic growth in agricultural sector, livestock, poultry and fisheries have to bear the burden. Professionals in India thus cannot ignore the demand of efficient and timely services. It is possible through the processes in place and continuous updating of knowledge, skills, competence besides, commitments of the professional groups in boosting animal production, productivity and product quality. The role of a Veterinarian in societal build up and its contribution in poverty alleviation and improving socio-economic betterment of small and landless livestock owners is becoming more and more demanding.

The serving veterinarian under the obligation of **'VETERINARY OATH'** which he takes at the time of obtaining registration under IVC Act, 1984 to continue to enhance his knowledge, skills and professional competence. The relevant portion of the OATH with reference to continuously updating knowledge & skills reads as **"I ACCEPT AS A LIFELONG OBLIGATION, THE CONTINOUS IMPROVEMENT OF MY PROFESSIONAL KNOWLEDGE AND COMPETENCE"**

Every professional thus is morally and socially bound to abreast himself with the latest knowledge and skills within the broad area of his domain and make use of these in discharge of his professional service delivery.

5.2.1 Institutional frame work for CVE

The department of Animal Husbandry, Dairying and Fisheries (DAHDF) Ministry of Agriculture, GOI, New Delhi has the responsibility to take measures to prevent the transmission or spread of diseases from one state to another. The DAHDF thus advices and support States and UT in formulation of policies and programs in the field of animal husbandry, dairying and fisheries.

After the creation of Indian Veterinary Council Act, 1984, the responsibilities to regulate veterinary practice is the primary responsibility of the VCI. The CVE was included in 10th plan document of the DAHDF with the purpose of implementing **'Professional Efficiency Development Programs'** in veterinary and animal sciences.

The secretary DAHDF in his recent presentation made in 2014 to the Prime Minister of India observed that there is shortage of trained Vets and Para-Vets. It was desired to start necessary short term skill development courses in consultation with the Veterinary Universities/ Colleges by utilizing their competent manpower. The department emphasized the need to organize CVE programs through the VCI. The council has also been advised to prepare course modules in the areas of relevance in the present day context. The modalities for the same are being worked out at the VCI level. The VCI has also to explore feasibility of associating with other agencies like the ICAR, SAUs, and national academy.

Though, many of the State Animal Husbandry departments have training institutes/schools which provide in-service training in the form of refresher courses, induction courses or courses on infertility management, A.I, vaccination and on other areas of importance. By and large these types are trainings are lecture based models with little emphasis on skill enhancements. In-fact, there is no structured CVE activities on regular basis that tone up professional skills and competence.

ICAR through its education division has many schemes/projects for competence enhancement of mainly teaching faculty. These include centers of advanced studies, summer/winter schools/short courses etc. There is however, very little for field functionaries.

Few SAUs/SVUs/Veterinary colleges have structured refresher courses to acquaint the field veterinarians with the latest developments. Further, to fulfill the mandatory requirement of certain research or transfer of technology projects, trainings are imparted to field functionaries and para-professionals. Hardly a few universities have structured training programs for the award of certificate or diploma on continuous basis.

The TNVASU, Chennai offers PG diploma in bio-informatics, veterinary laboratory diagnosis, companion animals practice and business management in animal and fisheries sciences. In addition the university offers diplomas in distance education online mode in 21 areas.

The IVRI also offers national diploma for field veterinarians in animal husbandry, biological products, preventive veterinary medicine, animal reproduction, equine husbandry, medicine & surgery, wild life and zoo management, poultry husbandry, feed and fodder technology and meat and meat processing technologies. Beside these, short term training courses are offered for field veterinarians and other research personals etc. Many other Universities and research Institutes organized training courses in specialized areas of their operations.

Open Universities: India is among the global leaders in providing distance learning through a network of Universities and distance educational institutions. The advantage of distance education over CVE is that the former cover mass education.

To expand the scope of trainings, National Academies like NAVS, NADS can become a viable partner in conducting CVE programs. The National Academy of Veterinary Sciences (I) can effectively take up centrally sponsored schemes on Professional Efficiency Development project for HR development in livestock sector.

There is a dire need for policy formulation and developing strategies for CVE. The VCI must take up this issue on priority basis and the Central Government (DAHDF), should allocate funds for operationalization of much needed CVE programs managed by Central and State agencies. In doing so,

It is worthwhile to study the relevance of CVE programs especially diploma or certificate courses being offered at institutes or universities for practicing veterinarians. There are very few takers of these programs.

N.B. The document on 'India, Human Resource development relevant to Veterinary Service Requirement. II. Continuing Veterinary Education in India: Challenges Ahead 'by Prof. (Dr) Rama Kumar V and Dr. Ajit Maru has been handy in preparation of this write up on CVE. This document may be referred for further details. (drramakumarv@yahoo.co.in) & (a.maru@planet.in)

❑❑❑

Chapter-6

Regulatory and Governance Mechanisms

This chapter deals with existing governance system and the complexity of inter-relationships with different regulatory authorities.

6.0 Introduction

Veterinary education is a state subject thus educational institutions are created and supported by the state governments. Thus for the purpose of creating institutions, impart education and grant degree is the sole function of the university. However, a qualified veterinary graduate becomes eligible to practice his/ her professional competence only when he possesses a recognized veterinary qualification and has sought registration with the VCI/ SVC. For this purpose the GOI had promulgated Indian Veterinary Council Act, 1984 (IVC Act) and established a statutory authority - the Veterinary Council of India (VCI) to regulate veterinary practice in states/ UT where and whenever the Act gets extended through the legislative provisions. Presently this Act has been extended throughout the country except in J&K.

To make the system operational the VCI brought out the following vital regulations in the first decade of its creation;

- VCI (Inspectors and Visitors) Regulations 1991
- VCI (Registration) Regulations 1992
- VCI (Standards of professional conduct, etiquette and code of ethics for veterinary practitioners') Regulations 1992
- VCI (Minimum standards of Veterinary Education-degree course (BVSc&AH) Regulations 1993 (MSVE), revised in 2008
- VCI (Election of President and Vice President) Regulations 1995

Beside these, it has also framed IVC rules in 1985 and several other guidelines which have been widely circulated from time to time.

In order to streamline veterinary education in the country, the VCI enforced implementation of MSVE, regulations, 1993 in veterinary colleges in India. Despite the fact, that states have accepted the onus to translate these regulations by appropriately providing needed support and most of the universities adopt the syllabus and academic regulation of the VCI in veterinary colleges at once. However, many of the states could not manage desired infrastructure and manpower as per the laid standards. Though, progressive improvisations in infrastructure at teaching institutions continued to occur over the time with the support from state governments and ICAR but most of the institutions have failed to touch desired level as per the VCI norms. Appreciable variability in infrastructure and human resource continues to exist between state to state and college to college. It is thus imperative that quality variability do exist between institutions.

Act is the basic/primary governance principle for any organization/system. Though, with the changing time, governance principles may require re-tuning, yet the IVC Act, 1984 has not lost its luster even today and this Act provides all necessary powers, authorities and tools to the authorities to make it relevant to fulfill the present day needs.

Acts or any regulations, rules, guidelines or any other governance tools are framed under the umbrella of the constitutional provisions. Thus, these are required to be read and interpreted to safeguard constitutional provisions.

The following constitutional provisions have direct relevance to veterinary education. Veterinary education is a state subject (7th schedule list II, S.No, 15). However, central government has been empowered to determine standards of higher education (7th schedule list- I, S.No.66). Relevant constitutional provisions are as under;

6.1 Article 246 7th Schedules of Indian constitution

6.1.1 List-1 Central issues

S.No. 66. Coordination and determination of standards in institutions of higher education or research and scientific and technical institutions.

Thus, under the provision of the IVC Act, 1984, the VCI has been empowered to determine the standards of veterinary education under Section 22 of the Act. In faithful subservience of the Act, the VCI laid has down 'Minimum Standards of Veterinary Education-degree course (BVSc&AH)' Regulations, 1993 which have been amended in 2008.

6.1.2 List II States issues

S.No. 15. Preservation, protection and improvement of stock and prevention of animal diseases, veterinary training and practice.

The aforesaid functions fall under the domains of the state governments. Veterinary institutions thus are created by the states for imparting education and training.

64. Offences against laws with respect to any of the matter in the list (under article 246, II schedule list-II-States).

State is empowered to take action against erring institution. Central govt. or the VCI is not empowered to resort to any direct action against any state controlled organizations.

The Constitutional provisions are very clear in defining the role of centre and state governments with respect to veterinary science sector. Role and responsibilities for the central and state governments have been clearly delineated whereby the central government has to determine the standards of education while the implementation of these rests with the universities/institutes. The VCI under section 19 and 20 is empowered to cause inspection of institution or college.

The very spirit behind promulgation of the IVC Act, 1984 was to regulate veterinary practice. Right type of veterinary education and trainings are pre-requisite and inseparable component of a practicing professional thus some definite provisions have been made in dealing with veterinary education in the Act. The provisions pertaining to veterinary education, so made, had no over-riding effect on the autonomy of the degree awarding institutions/ universities as well as the authorities of the states, since agricultural including veterinary education is a state subject. Constitutionally also the role of central government is *'Co-ordination and determination of standards in institutions for higher education or research and scientific and technical institutions'.*

Through, the power vested with the VCI, it has to prescribe the Minimum Standards of Veterinary education-degree course (MSVE) for the institutions to faithfully implement. Further, central govt. is empowered to grant recognition or withdraw recognition based upon the inspection/ visitation made by the VCI. It is thus implied that the veterinary institutions shall have to adhere to the prescribed standards at all its colleges/units otherwise their recognition of degree will be withdrawn by the central government after inspection/ visitation made by the VCI under section 21 of the Act. The graduates passing out from such institutions that are not listed in Schedule-1 of the Act or the recognition of institution or particular college has been withdrawn and entries' of such effects made in the Schedule-1 after the specified date, will not qualify for registration with the VCI/ State Councils and thus cannot practice as per section 29-30 of the Act. Privileges and rights of Registered Veterinary Practitioners have been spelt out in Section 29 & 30 of the IVC Act.

The relevant responsibilities of central authorities based upon the true spirit of the Act in context of Veterinary education are as under;

Central Govt. Dept. of Animal Husbandry, Dairying and Fisheries (DAHDF) has been empowered to grant recognition or withdrawal of recognition of degree on the advice of the VCI as per the authorities vested to it under IVC Act, 1984 to :

1. **Granting recognition** to the degree awarded by INSTITUTION (means any university or any other institution within or without India which grants degrees, diploma or licenses in veterinary sciences and animal husbandry) not included in the Schedule-1 (NEW INSTITUTIONS) under section 15 of the IVC Act.
2. **De-recognition/withdrawal of degree** awarded by institution or any of its college (EXISTING INSTUTIONS listed in Schedule-1) if found not adhering to the prescribed standards (MSVE, Regulations) framed under Section 22 of the Act. Section 21 of the IVC Act provides detail procedure for withdrawal of recognition.

The VCI is a professional statutory body to determine the status of the institution/college by inspection/ visitation and advice the central govt. on the adequacy of the standards or otherwise as per MSVE, Regulations. The DAHDF is the final dispersal authority to pass orders after consideration of the recommendations of the VCI by bringing amendment in the first Schedule of the IVC Act.

Other Sections of the Act that have bearings on veterinary education include Section 12 (constitutions of committees), 16, 17 (recognition of foreign degrees), 18 (to seeking information from institutions), 19 and 20 (inspection & visitation of institutions/colleges) are the supporting Sections to accomplish aforesaid two salient functions listed in S.No. 1 & 2.

Thus, the provisions of the Act clearly spell out the authorities of the central government, department of animal husbandry, dairying and fisheries and the VCI. If any college of an Institution/University whose degree is recognized and is enlisted in the First Schedule, does not conform to the prescribed MSVE, regulation, on inspections made under 19 or 20, the qualification for award of degree from such college shall be withdrawn as per the prescribed procedure laid down under section 21 of the Act.

6.2 The Functions and Responsibilities of Different Regulatory Authorities are Summarized below

6.2.1 State Government

- Full authority to enact governance principles through legislation or through administrative decisions for establishing and managing veterinary institution in the State.
- Make provisions in state budget
- Provide manpower and establishment cost to the institution.

6.2.2 Government of India (Central Government)

i. **VCI :** A body consistent of AH department, GOI created through the Act of parliament.

   Authorized body to regulate veterinary practice in India VCI also recommends to GOI to grant recognition to the degree awarded by the institution/ university through inspection for notification in the schedule of the IVC Act

   The VCI prescribe regulations and through these regulations it provides standards for

   - Academic norms
   - Course curriculum
   - Norms for space, building & departments, instructional farms; hospital complex etc.
   - Infrastructure-equipment
   - Manpower

ii. **ICAR :** A society registered under society Act (GOI) is the Apex body to guide, promote, partially aid, coordinate and regulate agricultural education including veterinary and animal sciences.

Support agricultural educational institutions including veterinary sciences through

'Development and Strengthening grant' to SAU's

- Provide research grant through various research schemes
- Establish KVK and other Transfer of Technology centers
- Make universities partners in education, research and extension programs
- Accreditation of institutions imparting agricultural educational programs.

6.2.3 University (SAU)*

- Custodian of veterinary college and its constituent unit
- Institute degree, diploma, licensing programs and award degrees, certifications etc.
- Apex body to delineate goals and objectives of the institutions through its academic bodies
- Oversee day to day management of its constituent colleges and create enabling environment
- Coordinate with state and central agencies to garner timely & appropriate support for the university.
- Translate effectively policies and programs of centre, state, statutary authorities and concerned scientific bodies etc.

**Universities are statutory authorities created under State Act. The State universities are recognized by the UGC under UGC Act, 1956*

Note: Lots of ups and downs have been witnessed during the last decade in managing the affairs of veterinary institutions. It has created disharmony between regulating and the implementing agencies. Taking cue from the past events, it is desired that the central govt. and VCI in particular draw out guidelines with respect to opening of new colleges, prescribe standard operative procedures (SOP) for inspections of institutions and other procedural details for better governance. It would be more prudent if such exercises are done in consultation/ collaborations with state agencies including universities.

The present governance mechanisms operative in the universities, especially personal policies, administrative procedures, financial management etc. are by and large dependent on state policies and as per the Act and provisions of the university. Besides these, the Model Act of ICAR, regulations of VCI and accreditation norms are imposing some compulsions in managing affairs of the universities. Since state government is custodian of the institutes established by it, general service rules and procedures are the guiding principles for the universities. Though, universities are supposed to be autonomous, but colonial rules and procedure, bureaucratic dominance, political interferences are some serious concern for university functioning. Ideally the Chancellor is the supreme authority for the university operations but the state governments keep check and control over the routine affairs of university activities. Too much mend- ling with the routine affairs of the universities/ colleges results into procedural delays and many a time useful activities/ projects are held up for obtaining administrative sanctions/ approval to the extent that these lose their relevance. It is irony of the situation that the age old financial rules are stumbling blocks for the developments and growth. The existing system has a great absorbing power for wasteful expenditure but one has to cross many hurdles even to incur petty essential expenses. Scientist gets disheartened to procure necessary items and at stages he has to compromise with the quality while following purchase procedures.

Delegation of power down the line is call of the day. Power is linked with responsibilities and accountability. Sharing of responsibilities makes decision making fast. Those universities/ organizations where there are structural arrangements of power sharing are high in the order of performance/ development. The universities are striving hard to streamline governance and financial management under the era of IT revolution. Many of the universities have/ are in the process of shifting to online financial management. The off campuses institutions which were under tremendous pressure to get financial sanctions or fund allocations are becoming comfortable with online system. Most of the universities have shifted to online advertisements/ application forms/ tender applications/ examination forms/ confidential examination activities etc. The governments should ensure liberal support to the universities for institution and installation of online support system and software development programs. Universities should be allowed to hire consultancy for the purpose. Extensive facilities for training of the staff on regular basis should be built in. Investments in modernization of IT technologies are bound to make system better responsive to the fast changing world order at a lesser cost and with faster pace. India needs to move with global pace to remain sustainable for developmental activities.

The State Universities have been/ are being created while adhering to the broad principles of ICAR Model Act for agricultural universities in India. For the purpose of establishing and managing the affairs of the SAUs or the universities carved out from agricultural universities (veterinary, horticulture and fishery sciences), the Model Act is the guiding force. Though the states have to modify some of the provisions of the Model Act to accommodate states policies and programs but there exists wide variations between states with respect to basic governance principles which is making difficult for ICAR to bring uniformity in SAUs. Most visible variations include; composition, power and authorities of BOM/ Executive Council, manner of appointment and tenure of VC, nomenclature of university officers/ faculty, provision of affiliation etc. In some universities there are too many public representatives or large proportion of internal members on the BOM that questions the very spirit of autonomy or decision making.

Another area of concern is recruitments in the universities. There is complete stagnation in SAUs/ SVUs to recruit faculty through lateral entry at senior positions of associate professors, professors, deans, directors etc. Open advertisement and selection on the post have become merely a formality as hardly any fresh talent is inducted to man such positions. In- fact talent hunt, mobility of scientist, induction of talent through open recruitment, competitiveness, reducing inbreeding etc. are less visible. In true sense recruitments have become in-house manage-mental system. Our recruitment and promotion policies by and large are not conducive for growth.

A study in this context may be commissioned to compile detail scenario of the country. There is a need to accept the ground realities and evolve a system that should be able to address to the progressive programs. The ICAR and the VCI may deliberate on this subject with the Vice Chancellors and other related organizations and draw a workable plans to ensure progressive policies conducive for growth.

□□□

Chapter-7

Private Veterinary Education & 'Public Private Partnership' (PPP) In India

7.1 Introduction

Keeping in view global developments taking place in multidimensional sectors of veterinary and animal sciences, and in order to built competent human resource to manage the commitments effectively; heavy investments are required to be pumped in education sector. Governments (center and states) on their own are unable to cope up with the upsurge of national demands in a fast changing scenario of global competitiveness. It is thus imperative that to built up and expand infrastructure and provide greater financial access to revamp higher education, massive support from private sector is the need of the hour. Ernst and Young- FICCI report emphasis **that Public Private Partnership (PPP) could be an effective mechanism for much needed private sector investment in higher education system without diluting the regulatory oversight of the government and other regulatory agencies**. The PPP is one of the many possible ways to manage developments on massive scale.

Government is conscious of the fact that enabling environment has to be created to attract private players to become partners in the process of development. Indian experiences of 'Public Private Partnership' (PPP) in other sectors have been a mixed bag. National highways, Railways, Power and other commercially viable sectors are the areas where government is attracting partners from private sector, and such partnerships have shown encouraging trends. However, by and large higher education has been one of the areas that remained greatly untapped. Though, some fragmentary attempts for developing partnerships in commercialized based agricultural and allied sectors (plants and animal genomics, transgenic plants, animal & fishes, food processing technologies, vaccine production and its quality control, embryo technologies, agri-business and development of agro-processing units etc.) in a bid to enhance productivity through application of newer biotechnology tools for boosting agriculture for the service of mankind have shown positive trends. However, PPP in its true perspective is yet to be conceptualized and effectively operationalized in establishing educational institutions in PPP mode with requisite potentials to unify educational programs. By and large education imparted through private sector is misconceived as PPP. Education through private sector in veterinary education is new addition to the age old education being imparted and managed mainly through public sector organizations such as state agricultural system. Despite the fact that the central government and the VCI are conscious for the need to develop oversight mechanism to monitor and regulate educational standards in private institutions but it is yet to develop a workable system for the same. Unified approach on the part of the government and regulatory organizations in planning, execution and monitoring education system in totality is a daunting challenge. It of course is required to be understood that government must develop open door policy and ensure that private partners are attracted to share the burden of filling up the vital gaps in what we have and what is required.

7.2 Present status of Higher Education in India

It would be worthwhile to present projections of higher education in India before dwelling specifically on veterinary education.

Today in India only 12.4% of the eligible candidates enroll for higher education as against 50-60% in US and Canada. India has about 700 universities with around 35,000 colleges having a total capacity to enroll 17 million students which is grossly inadequate. Access to higher agricultural education is much less and deficient in terms of quality output, lack requisite minimum standards, enrollment capacity and availability of competent human resource. Graduate enrolment ratio (GER) is skewed to the tune of 19.4% in India which is only 1/2 to that of world average. In advanced countries like US and Canada GER ratio is 50-60%. The 12th plan considered level of incremental expansion in GER by 10%. Extrapolating similar trends in agricultural sector more and more institutions of global order are required to be created. The National Knowledge Commission (NKC) headed by Sam Patroda has recommended establishment of 1500 universities in India as a long term goal. However, this gigantic task has to be taken up in phased manner. The NKC also envisages breaking up of existing large universities into smaller and to permit autonomous colleges to expand into universities. Thus carving out of veterinary and animal sciences universities out of the state agricultural universities could be considered a desirable step in this direction. Government of India has allocated 1545 billion for higher education in the 12th five year plan. The Planning Commission has identified a resource gap of Rs. 2.2 trillion. It is unlikely that the government alone can fulfill this gap to build much needed infrastructure for higher education in near future. It is also a fact that there is an unequal outlay of resources for higher education across the Indian states which is creating disharmony. Government resources are reaching saturation level to take up such a heavy task of establishing more and more quality Institutions. Thus there is a need to rope private sector to pump in heavy investments on regular basis. However, in doing so public sector will have to take a step forward in developing cohesive relationship and developing strong bondages, mutual trust and reposing faith in each other. Private sector should also to assure for long term commitments and adhering to the prescribed standards and quality assurance norms. The programs should be market driven and drawn by joint mechanisms involving both public and private organizations. PPP is required to be capitalized on mutual strength to accelerate the progress of educational developments.

The concept of 'Public Private Partnership in Veterinary Education in India' is required to be clearly understood. **Privatization and public private partnership are not synonym. Partnership stands for a cohesive relationship, sound bondage, mutual trust and faith in each other.** Further entering into public private partnership is in no way dilute or infringe on the regulatory mechanisms or create any form of unhealthy competitiveness. Instead, the basic philosophy of PPP calls for potential mechanisms to attract private sector. Further, the wisdom and experiences of private player would help in creating viable models to assist the government. The government may facilitate suitable land and other fixed infrastructure for the private sector to build necessary and viable models to complement the efforts of the government in growth and developmental programs. It is also required to be ensured that there is periodic monitoring of standards and quality assurance of education through national and international accreditation bodies.

7.3 Present Status and Developments in Veterinary Sector

The veterinary educational institutes are passing through a serious crisis of human resource. More than 60% of the colleges are not even maintaining 50% of the requisite manpower in numerical strength thereby greatly hampering quality standards in imparting educational training. Further quality research output and transfer of technological programs from these colleges are out of reach with the available faculty. Lately privatization of veterinary education is making headway in the country. As of today 10 private colleges have been established (7 in Rajasthan, one each in UP, Punjab and Haryana) but somehow these are yet to be inducted in the main stream. Institutions coming up in private sector are expected to remain under privileged owing primarily to the fact that governance system in vogue has its boundaries encompassing only public sector. As the situation that stands today, the role of private sector as partner in the process of development is negligible. Dr. M.S. Swaminathan committee on Agricultural Education on the issues of improving education in private institutions to enable ICAR to maintain uniform academic standards emphasized a need to enforce structural changes in private institutions so that these institutions also compliment the efforts of the government in discharging the committed and collective responsibility in nation building. In order to achieve this, it was suggested to provide some 'Development grants' for updating of libraries, laboratory equipments and farms and for establishment of educational technology cell to potential private institutes.

Prof. A.L. Choudhary, former president of the VCI, in his address at the second convocation at the Karnataka Veterinary , Animal and Fishery Science University in 2005 emphasized that " The situation demands that as in the case of medical, technical, management education, private entrepreneur need to be motivated to participate in veterinary education and research." He also exhibited his concern over the existing number of veterinarians around 42,000 as against the need for 72,000. Such situation is bound to have a negative impact on the implementation and success of research and development programs. He further stressed the need for public private partnership in veterinary education mainly quantity of education and suggesting framing and enforcing effective regulations. Further, salient recommendations emerging on the subject under discussion from the National Seminar on 'Strategies for strengthening of Veterinary Education and practice sector' held at Hyderabad on 13-14 Dec, 2008 are.

"In order to meet the requirement of qualified veterinary practitioners by the services sector, more veterinary colleges both in the public as well as private sectors should opened and the admission intake of the existing colleges may be increased subject to strict fulfillment of the relevant VCI regulation in force from time to time. For enhancement of the admission intake of students in the existing colleges, these should be strengthened proportional to the increase. Further, as many private entrepreneurs have started showing interest in opening new colleges, the possibilities of public private partnership in opening new colleges should be explored to encourage their participation in the development of veterinary sector".

With the increased demand for veterinary graduates to meet the requirement of the service, education and research sectors, there has been an exponential increase in the proposals for opening of new veterinary colleges both in the public as well as private sector. While this private partnership in the veterinary education sector is a welcome step, it is imperative that a robust regulatory mechanism is put in place to ensure quality of education at these institutions since their opening. The requirement of infrastructure and teaching manpower in private colleges meant only for imparting undergraduate education would have to be worked out separately in view of their specific objectives.

As the information on the actual requirement of manpower in education and service sectors in terms quality and quantity shall be crucial in developing strategies for strengthening of these sectors, a study should be commissioned to assess the need on a short and long term basis. The mandate of this exercise should also encompass on the manpower requirements of veterinary colleges in private sector in light of their specific objective of undergraduate teaching alone.

7.4 Need for Retuning of Veterinary Education System

Veterinary profession used to be mainly under public domain and graduates were primarily gaining entry into govt. line departments mainly as Veterinary officer and extension specialists. This trend is progressively changing owing to diversification in job profiles of professionals working in livestock sector and thus there is a need to re-tune the entire system.

Out of approximately 40,000 Veterinary professionals position, around 75-80% are in govt. jobs and 10% in teaching and scientific organizations. A small segment of Veterinary professional are in co-operative and NGO sector (like NDDB, milk unions, agro-industries, Insurance, banks, pharmaceuticals, food processing industries etc). Only a few hundred are self-employed as practitioners, farm owners, veterinary management etc. Traditionally there was a general perception that veterinarians are only meant to care for or treat sick and injured animals. However, **today's veterinarians have to shoulder wider responsibilities in diversified spectrum of social system. Ensuring food safety, public health, meat inspection, wild life conservation and environmental protection, animal welfare, biotechnology, quarantine and defense against bioterrorism, quality assurance and export of food products etc are the areas where veterinarian is expected to play his role at the centre stage.**

The relationship between human health, animal health and the ecosystem are the inseparable component of social set up. Bio safety tools, conservation of natural recourses, food securities, nutritionally balanced diet have become integral component of job roaster for veterinarian. Vital component of newer challenges and responsibilities are mainly under the domain of co-operative sector and therefore in order to address these effectively and speedily, cohesive approach between public -private sector and entrepreneurs his becoming time demanding.

Presently by and large graduates are undergoing almost stereotype course curricula and trainings. It is not that programs are not being updated but to match the developments taking place nationally or globally, course curricula are periodically reviewed and modified. However, owing to the system being almost water jacketed, graduates are being produced with almost identical knowledge and skills. Though on one side, core basic knowledge and skills are prerequisite for a veterinary graduate but apart from it there is a need to give flexibility to the graduating students to undergo specialized training in the areas of his/her interest. Along with it, additional knowledge acquisition processes even across the faculty/institution should be built in the system. May be, the number of veterinary graduates entering in corporate, industrial sector are low but looking to the recent trends, their demand is on the rise. By and large their performance output in private sector may have been satisfactory, but it is time for us to introspect as to how far the knowledge and skills they have acquired while undergoing courses are useful to them or their organizations in their diversified career endeavors. Let some institution like VCI/ICAR sponsor a study to find out the usefulness of course contents in career built up of a graduate. It may not be astonishing, that in certain situations there is no match between what has been taught vis-à-vis what is required in job pursuits. The outcome of such a study would provide guidelines for bringing out a strategic shift to the existing system.

Industrial houses are spending large amount of money for the human resource development in shaping the personality of its employee to suit to their requirements. Time and money spent in shaping a raw graduate could be minimized if some structural changes as per the requirements of employer are made in the curricular planning and its execution during degree course. This would possible only when public-private mechanisms are interwoven in a common thread so that demands of the user agencies are rightfully met with the availability of competent professionals to cater their specific needs.

The basic objectives and the primary goals of institutions both under public or private are the same. Further each institute has to ensure for quality output and abide by the defined policy framework. Unless and until institutions are given parallel status, growth and development would not yield desired dividends. It is to be understood that there should be equality of principles for academic management, academic governance and academic operational freedom for any institutions irrespective of its being in public or private sector. Under the changing scenario, metamorphic approach is needed right from conceptualization stage to its final execution, so as to bring transformation toward making our system vibrant and productive, especially in producing professionals, who are competent, self-reliant and possess the capabilities to swiftly adjusting to the changing environment. It calls for restructuring of educational programs.

7.5. Restructuring and Delivery of Educational Programs

7.5.1 All programs running under PPP mode should also address to the needs of private sector as well. Further, their input on a common forum would be bilaterally beneficial.

7.5.2 There should be provisions to have proper representation from private sector in academics, planning and management bodies.

7.5.3 Sharing of facilities and expertise should be encouraged.

7.5.4 Faculty from private sector should be given equal opportunity for competence enhancement. Further, scientific or technocrat cadre from private institute should structure hands on training programs in their areas of their expertise for the faculty from public sector. Public sector partners should be given limited access to their operational/production units as and when need arises.

7.6 Policy Changes Proposed

7.6.1 There is a need to bring policy changes to facilitate developing strong and sustainable bondages between public and private sectors. Such changes would call for amendments/modifications in governance tools viz By-Laws, Act, regulations, guiding principles etc. State university's Act should be synchronous between different organizations and fully satisfy defined policy frame work.

7.6.2 Centre-State coordination for unified approach should be clearly spelt out.

Institutions have been/are being created by the state governments independent to the advice of VCI, ICAR or central govt. In order to foster these institutions they are made constituent units of the state agricultural or veterinary universities. Private veterinary colleges though have been established but no clear-cut policy or guidelines have been laid down by the central or state governments in this context. In view of this, lot of confusion prevails. Thus no defined procedures are being followed in granting permission to establish veterinary colleges in private sector. Even in SAU system, institutions are created with no set pattern. There is need to develop Standard Operative Procedures (SOP) for opening new colleges.

7.6.3 Standard Operative Procedure needed

With the changing scenario of veterinary education, there is a need to delineate Standard Operative Procedure (SOP) and sound operation of veterinary colleges. However, the participation of the private sector in veterinary and AH education has become a subject for debate and is required to be seen with objectivity. A suitable mechanism to regulate and monitor the education in private colleges also needs to be in place. The existing mechanism of monitoring of the colleges/institutions gives more emphasis toward physical facilities rather than evaluating standards of physical assets in commensuration with the quality assurance.

7.6.4 Center-State Coordination

It would be desirable to clearly delineate and define the centre-state coordinating mechanisms for smooth functioning. Moreover, a cohesive approach and delineation of authority and responsibilities between professional bodies, technocrats and bureaucrats need serious consideration for efficiency and vibrancy in decision making process. In conclusion, concrete steps are required to be initiated by the regulatory authorities to ensure effective participation of the private sector in providing constructive support to the public sector for filling the wide gap between demand and supply pertaining to HRD developmental programs and to meet other primary needs of the profession.

The following steps are suggested for closer coordination in public and private sector organizations in order to enforce needed reforms-

7.6.4.1 Change of mind set

The foremost criterion in developing effective partnership between the institutions is change of mindset. Till lately only public sector organizations were in existence and there is general perception that imparting education is the domain of public sector organizations only. Today the scenario has changed. Govt. has allowed establishment of private institutions and their mandated functions in the reference to graduate output are no different than their counterpart in public sector. These institutions are affiliated to the universities (SAUs/SVUs) for the purpose of academic management, course contents, examinations etc. Thus the universities have full regulatory control over the academic affairs of these affiliating units but what is required to be understood by the organizations is that managing the affairs of the educational units (constituents or affiliating), the parameter of assessing the quality of educational programs should remain the same. Let affiliating unit be given operational freedom in managing the affair of the institute. They of course should not be given leverage to deviate/sidetrack the hierarchial structure and laid down governance principles of the university.

7.6.4.2 Sharing of information and expertise

There is need for developing system for sharing of information and resources (resource here implies only to expertise, laboratories, library, farm facilities etc.). Electronic information system could be an effective linkage tool. Colleges can effectively co-operate and coordinate in developing information relevant to animal health, animal production and the prevention and control of animal diseases. Sharing of information will be of mutual benefit in focusing on teaching/learning environment. It is also established fact that individual college cannot marshal the resources to build the strength in all the disciplines to the level of excellence. Viable arrangement of sharing of expertise is thus called for. Further, successful research effort today, more than ever before, depends on group research rather than individual efforts. This would be possible in developing inter-institutional linkages.

7.6.4.3 Platform for frequent interactions

Some structural arrangement can be made for the scientists to interact in issues of common interest. Thorough as per the university's Act and Statues, various bodies have been defined viz. committee of courses, faculty academic council etc. yet while formulating policies and programs pertaining to educational reforms, university/college can develop platforms to seek input from private institutions.

7.6.4.4 Healthy Competition

The primary goal of an institution is to produce quality human resource. Every institute must strive to achieve the goal. Let the institute compete for academic excellence. Besides the student competing internally, they should be exposed to inter institutional competitions. Universities should develop some mechanism in this context. Likewise students must get opportunities to compete for co-curricular and extracurricular activities.

In Conclusion it is emphatically stated that under the changing scenario, metamorphic approach is needed to bring transformation toward making our system more vibrant & productive, especially in producing professionals, who are competent, self-reliant and possess the capabilities to swiftly adjusting to the changing environment. Change of mind set, coupled with coordinated efforts, public-private partnership & critical assessment of input to anticipated output as well as outcome analysis are the key component of the developmental processes. Both central and state governments, the scientific organizations, academies and associations, the universities & colleges, industrial houses and other stake holders should work in tandem to revamp the system for faster and meaningful developments of this sector.

Industrial and private sector organizations are very selective in inducting personals. Their preferences are not merely on the degree or qualification one is possessing, but the competence, skills, ability and attitude candidate possess suiting to the job pursuits. In such situations veterinary graduates are competing with dairy, agriculture, food sciences, fisheries and many other technocrats from allied sectors. Thus unlike jobs in AH departments in public sector earmarked specifically for veterinary graduate, for him to enter into private sector he has to sail through the ocean to prove his superiority.

□□□

Chapter-8

Lower Education

Effective delivery of professional services in veterinary and animal sciences is essentially dependent on support services (Minor veterinary service/Para-professional service). Professional expertise services go a begging if proper support system is not built in appropriately. It has been identified that para-veterinarians play increasingly important role of in livestock service delivery.

Massive work force is required to manage entire spectrum of livestock related activities in the country. In order to meet the requirements for not only of public sector organizations, but also many of those are attached to non-governmental organizations like private animal farms, industrial houses, practitioners, entrepreneurs etc, the VCI has identified their role and responsibilities. Further, states have to delineate frame work of their job profile and notify these in the official gazette under which they are expected to perform.

The IVC Act, 1984 under section 30 prescribe that **no person other than a Registered Veterinary Prectitioner,** Shall

"Practice veterinary medicine in any State"

Provided that the state government may, by order, permit a person holding diploma or certificate of veterinary supervisor, stockman or stock assistant (by whatever named called) issued by the Director of Animal Husbandry (by whatever named called) of any state or any veterinary institution in India, to render under the supervision and direction of a registered veterinary practitioner, minor veterinary services.

'Minor Veterinary services' means the rendering of preliminary veterinary aid, like vaccination, castration and dressings of wounds, and such other types of preliminary aids or treatment of such ailments as the State Government may, by notification in the official Gazette specify in this behalf. Every state ought to have made such notification for proper operation of their services under minor veterinary services.

In subservience to the provision of the IVC Act, every state government has organized structured training programs, to equip the para-professionals in order to acquire competence in the identified areas as notified in the gazette.

There are hundreds of Lower education schools/institutes/ polytechnics offering diploma/certificate courses to produce Para-Professionals in livestock and dairy sector. Maharashtra alone has 97 schools while Rajasthan has 65 such institutes and Andhra has 10 polytechnics. There is wide variability between the numbers of such schools, academic regulations, and entry level qualification and governance system of managing these schools/institutes. The Maharashtra produces around 1500 diploma holder every year against admission capacity of around 3500. Likewise, in Rajasthan with annual intake capacity of 3250 output is around 15-1600. It is necessary to exhibit concerns (where ever these exist) on over production of para-professionals with sub-optimal training which would be detrimental to the profession at large. Despite the dependency on the services of para-professionals, there are serious concerns over the quality output. The other disturbing trends that are generally seen are that they go beyond their service boundaries and perform services for which they are neither authorized nor equipped or trained for. It is thus of vital significance that there should be a strong monitoring and regulatory system in order to effectively make use of their services and restrict them to their jurisdiction of responsibilities. It is feared that at times there could be unhealthy competitions with the degree holders in delivery of professional services which do not fall within job pursuits of para-professionals. Hence, a definite policy in this direction is called for.

Although, every state has a responsibility to manage creation of institutions, structuring program, delineating the charter of duties and responsibilities, eligibility criteria, duration of program, course curriculum, academic regulations, monitoring and evaluation and manage mental control of these institutions etc yet in order to bring some amount of unanimity across the states, the VCI may put forth very broad guiding principles in the form of regulations. In Rajasthan, entry qualification for 2 year diploma is 10+2. The identified skills required include taking temperature, providing preliminary veterinary aids for analgesic and antipyretic in case of fever and pain, perform A.I, vaccination, dressing of wounds, castration of male by castrator, collection of samples and spray for ecto-parasitic control. Other states also have notified the desired skills of para-professionals.

Presently, the lower educational institutions have been created as constituent units of the university/AH departments or affiliated units created and managed by private organizations. In two of the states of the country viz Maharashtra that has 97 lower education schools, created under private sector and Rajasthan having 65 schools are managed by the respective State Veterinary Universities. Andhra has 10 AH polytechnic and one in fishery Science while Kerala offers diploma in poultry production, laboratory technology and dairy production. It also offers certificate course in wild life management and established a distance learning centre. Though, at MAFSU, a post of Associate Dean, Lower education exists while at RAJUVAS, the COE has been entrusted the responsibilities to manage these schools yet there is no defined system available in most of the states to manage these schools. To cater to the responsibilities in managing the academic activities of large number of schools spread across the state, lot of time is being devoted to oversee the academics at these schools which definitaly hamper into the activities of higher education.

Thus in order to effectively manage the lower education, it would be prudent to create a separate Directorate of lower education within or without the university.

From the national perspective, the VCI Act, 1984 created a provision for certain personal holding diploma or certificate of veterinary supervisor, stockman, stock assistant, compounders, veterinary assistant, pharmacists, livestock assistant etc. to render MINOR VETERINAY SERVICES under the supervision of a registered veterinary practitioner (RVP).

With the expansion of livestock sector, a veterinarian has to be associated with multi fold responsibilities of managing health care, breeding, feeding, management of livestock and transfer of technological practices and the para-professional also are bound to support registered veterinary practitioner (RVP) for added responsibilities. The Govt. of Andhra had constituted an expert committee with the purpose to provide a better basis for the planning, monitoring and evaluation through a well considered regulatory frame work in managing the affairs of such support system. The major objectives were to propose basic definition for Minor Veterinary Services/ Minor Veterinary Dispensations in specific context of AP, to shortlist context/ skills for differently qualified para-vets and develop course contents etc.

The expert committee constituted by Andhra Government recommended the State to adopt the following definition for 'Minor Veterinary Service'

"Basic Veterinary interventions, dispensations and livestock extension (as specified in schedule I, II, III)* provided by trained and certified personnel, other than registered veterinary practitioners to support livestock, health and production.

*Schedule I	All general extension and fodder development services (which require basic orientation training)
*Schedule II	All services that require systematic skill development and guidance of a registered veterinary practitioner
*Schedule III	All services that require advanced training and supervisory guidance of a registered veterinary practitioner

The author is not conversant with the status of lower education in different states of the country but decidedly every state must be having some system of operation of lower educational programs that are in commensuration to cater to the needs of the state on one hand and adherence to the defined norms for running the program on the other. It however, is suggested that there should be a broad frame work under which the state can delineate its policies and programs. States can take advantage from the AP model (Reference may be made to the Research Report 'Minor Veterinary Service in Andhra Pradesh: Stake holder consultation & Expert Group Deliberation CALPI RR Nr.05-08, Oct, 2005).

The VCI whose prime responsibility under the provision of the Act is to regulate veterinary practice but it still has to go a long way in regulating practice effectively across the country. It is desired that mechanisms are required to be developed to ensure optimum standards of veterinary institutions dealing with animal health care and regulating practice including minor veterinary services more vigorously. There should be more frequent interactions between state agencies with the VCI to device meaningful modalities/ stretagies to transform much needed changes.

❑❑❑

Part-II
Invited Articles

The primary aim of the veterinary educational institutions is to build a professional character that must have inherent capacity to deliver in the overall ambit of the acquired qualification. In order to do so, broadly the system has to deliver effectively under the broad umbrella of two dimensions (i) animal husbandry practices ie breeding, feeding, housing, management with the view to boost production. These practices would become meaningful only when these are effectively transferred to the welfare of the end user-the farming community and (ii) animal health care (prevention and control of diseases) of animals including wild animals and birds.

After completion of foundation courses at the initial stages of degree course, the students have to learn to apply knowledge and skills in holistic manner to bring out meaningful interpretations that requires ILFC and TVCC- the two primary units that provide learning and training platforms for the students to acquire professional competence.

Keeping the importance of these two essential pre-requisites, experts' inputs on vital components of ILFC and TVCC have been incorporated. Ensuing chapters 9 to 13 deals on these issues.

Chapter-9

Instruction Livestock Farm Complex (ILFC)

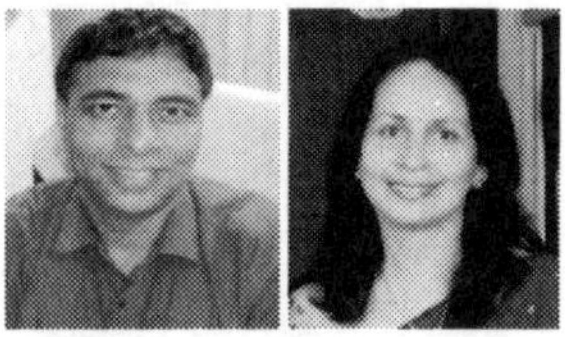

Prof. (Dr) VISHNU SHARMA & Prof. (Dr) SANJITA SHARMA*

DEAN

Post Graduate Institute for Veterinary Education and Research, Jaipur

**Professor and Head, Department of LPM*

9.1 Preamble

Though, livestock (animal) farms remained an integral component of veterinary colleges/institutions but the VCI for the first time emphasized the need of establishing an independent unit of ILFC having as status of a full fledged department of a veterinary college as per the revised 'Minimum Standards of veterinary Education-degree course (BVSc&AH), Regulations', 2008. The provision reads as under 'The instructional Livestock Farm Complex shall be a separate unit in every veterinary college under the independent charge of a faculty member of the rank of a Professor with specialization in any of the production subjects'. **The basic philosophy of having a separate Instruction Livestock Farm Complex (ILFC) in VCI curriculum was to equip veterinary students with requisite skills apart from knowledge gained during the various subject courses taught in the curriculum of B.V.Sc. & A.H.**

9.2 Mandate & Objectives

The existing mandate of ILFC under VCI focused towards imparting teaching ***in rearing of livestock species*** including poultry and hands ***on training of the students*** on the overall farm practices of livestock management including cleaning, feeding, watering, grooming, milking, routine health care, record keeping, sanitation, housing and fodder production etc.

The ILFC has been treated largely as a practical training course of LPM subject, whereas, looking towards the expectations of the society, the ILFC should ***inculcate and equip students with required skills*** necessary for safe and clean production of milk, meat, egg, wool and other animal products required by a cross section of society. Therefore, a veterinary student should expose to all backward and forward linkages of animal product so as he/she have sufficient capacity, confidence and command to be an ***entrepreneur***.

9.3 Practices

The major areas of training includes so far are Cattle, Buffalo, Sheep, Goat, Pig, Horse, Rabbit, Poultry and Fish farming along with fodder production and Grassland management. Largely, emphasis is given to back ward linkages and mainly for rearing practices leading to the deficiency in processing, marketing skills that could not effectively translate in entrepreneurship. Following are few areas which needs sufficient space in ILFC model:

9.3.1 Diversified animal farming

ILFC should also include various types of integrated livestock farming models according to the regional requirement. Further, veterinary students needs good exposure for poultry other than chickens and broilers such as turkeys, ducks, geese, quails, emu, ostriches, Aqua, Seri and Pisci culture enterprises so as to promote them to apply their veterinary knowledge background for up-scaling the value chain processes.

9.3.2 Animal Feed Processing

The ILFC should cater essentially animal feed processing unit as an important back ward linkage. The student should have hands on training for preparing various types of feeds ranging from aqua, pet, poultry and dairy feeds in different delivery forms like mash, pellet, biscuits, crumbles, block, bricks, mineral mixture etc. This sector bears tremendous demand for veterinarians to emerge as entrepreneur and business personnel.

9.3.3 Animal Product Processing

The concept of value chain and value addition needs to be inculcating in the minds of students and for this, ILFC curriculum should extend beyond production but up to processing. ILFC should have small milk, meat, egg and wool processing units where student can himself evaluate the complete value chain of the product and can be conceptualized with the concept of ***Safe Product*** rather than mere ***product*** only.

9.3.4 New Production Systems

Students need to practice organic livestock production, integrated livestock production systems, Non-conventional livestock farming system, sustainability and environmental protection etc to be coherent with global mandate. Facilities of vermi composting, bio digester, bio-gas plant for power generation, waste management and recycling etc.

9.3.5 Marketing, Business & Entrepreneurship

The students should provide opportunity to explore study, negotiate and market the product. Such steps will create real exposure to the students regarding real situation in the market, profits, consumer choice, marketing chain, cost-benefit etc.

9.4 Participatory Departments

Livestock Production and Management, Animal Nutrition, Livestock Production & Technology, Animal Breeding & Genetics, Poultry Science, Veterinary Extension Education, Veterinary Public Health and Production Physiology are essential participatory components of ILFC. Further services of Agronomist to manage fodder production would prove beneficial.

9.5 Credit & Course Induction

Presently, as per VCI norms, only two courses of ILFC taught in II year but students at this level are still studying basic courses and there placement at ILFC is not very appropriate. It would be more prudent if the existing courses (LFP 211 and LFP 221) should be shifted to third year of the degree course as (LFP 311 and LFP 321). Beside these, two more courses for (i) LFP 411- LS Product processing & Packaging and (ii) LFP-421 Entrepreneurship and marketing should be introduced.

9.6 Basic Layout of Instructional Units

9.6.1 Production Section

This section includes farms of various species. It is clarified that the instructional farm are non-commercial unit.

- Large ruminant section: Cattle & Buffalo farm (Minimum 50 adult animals with followers)
- Small ruminant section: Sheep & Goat Farm: (Minimum 50-100 animals in each farm)
- Piggery farm (minimum 50-100 animals)- based on regional need
- Equine unit (Minimum 2 Horse)
- Poultry Farm (Layers, broilers, hatchery and sample stock of other birds-quails, turkey, emu etc.)
- Fish Pond
- Rabbit farm
- Bee keeping
- Animals of regional interest
- Fodder production & management : 20-50 acres of land sufficient to meet the requirement of fodder for the livestock. At hilly tracts or where non productive and terrain lands are available, minimum area required for fodder production may be suitably modified. It has to be kept in mind that fodder production should be viable venture for the college and not a liability of any form on the institution.

9.6.2 Animal Feed Section

Pellet making Machine, Feed block, Grinder, Mixture, UMMB, Mineral Mixture, Silo pits etc.

9.6.3 Processing Section

Should be equipped to have Milk and Meat processing plants, Modern slaughter house and abattoir, egg processing unit etc.

9.7 Student Involvement

The students should be given complete task of producing, processing and marketing of desired product with all backward and forward logistics. There may be groups of students targeted for task and suitable modalities should develop so that students can be partner in business profit and decision making. Post Graduate students should also essentially be placed and rotates in different units of ILFC and may be given task for close monitoring of ILFC. The post graduate program in production subjects should have more credits for practical aspects of ILFC and it should stretch at least for one year with an opportunity of selecting Elective enterprise according to choice and facilities available.

The concept of ILFC in veterinary science education system is worth appreciating and caters the great demand and expectations of society. However, in present form it is not capable of producing vet as an independent entrepreneur, corporate, managers and supporting element in value chain of livestock business. The industry is ready to take veterinary, provided he is equipped with minimum required skills and vision. The involvement of industry should also explore by the institutions for regionally important enterprises.

Shift is required in basic approach, execution practices and desired outcome of ILFC in a way that it will become the backbone of the whole veterinary curriculum.

9.8 Staff Requirement

1. HOD, ILFC (Professor Rank)-1
2. Farm Manager (Associate Professor Rank)-2
3. Assistant Professor–5 (LPM-2 and one each in Nutrition, Breeding, LPT, VPH and Agronomy)
4. Manager Farm operation-2
5. Farm Assistant-2
6. Animal attendants-4
7. Farm labour (As per work load)

9.9 Epilogue

The ILFC is an essential functional unit of veterinary colleges. Though, the colleges have created ILFC to fulfill the statutory needs of the VCI, but in true sense neither its role has been properly conceptualized nor it is fully operational at most of the institutions. The ILFC does offer two non credit courses, serve as 'hands on training' unit but there is a need to induct two more courses for LPM, Nutrition, LPT, Marketing and Interns undergo training in internship programs yet facilities and expertise available are not appropriately utilized. To enhance the utility of ILFC, institutes can take advantage of offering training as a part of continuing educational programs for competence enhancement of academic as well as service personals. Such an approach will enhance the viability of the institute, help in resource generation and shall be able to effectively make use of the available facilities.

□□□

Chapter-10

An Ideal Approach to Extension Education at Veterinary Educational Institutions

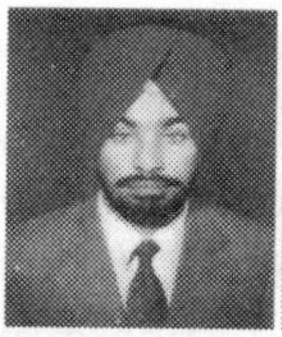 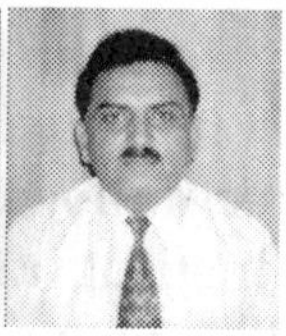

JASWINDER SINGH* AND H K VERMA**
*District Extension Specialist (Vety.Sci.)** Professor
Department of Veterinary and Animal Husbandry Extension Education
Guru Angad Dev Veterinary & Animal Sciences University, Ludhiana

10.1 Preamble

Livestock is an important sub sector of Indian agriculture economy and plays a multifaceted role in providing livelihood support to the rural population. Livestock sector apart from contributing to national economy, provides employment generation opportunities, asset creation, cope up the uncertainties of crop production and it becomes a dependable safeguard against crop failure, social and financial security. Recent trend shows that the growth in livestock sector has been at faster pace than crop sector. The growth of value added livestock products and byproducts has been exceedingly good, however, the demand for livestock products is galloping in coming years owing to the fact that there is greater awareness towards public health concerns, better shelf life of the products, availability of dependable cold chain for efficient storage, changes in lifestyle, increased work pressure and better purchasing power. The future strategy for achieving targeted livestock production should be on productivity enhancement and this would be possible only through the initiatives taken together by knowledge generation and dissemination agencies to the stakeholders. To hit the target of growth rate of 6-7% per annum there is a dire need to prepare state wise livestock and dairy development policies and plans. A functional extension education wing in the university/colleges need to be created where hitherto not created and needs to be strengthened in terms of infrastructure, qualified competent manpower and appropriate support system where it exists. To match the demand and supply of livestock products in the future, latest technologies and recommended practices are needed to be disseminated to the livestock farmers so that they can improve the animal performance as well as improve hygienic production and storage of livestock products. To manage these vast and integrated extension services are needed.

In an integrated system of teaching, research and extension, education gets the highest priority followed by research while extension education or transfer of technological practices are placed at the bottom in most of the teaching institutions. Is it not an irony of the situation that not more than 15-20% technologies generated are transferred to the end users? Further, very low percentage of these have actually been adopted by the farming community.

The importance of extension education and extension activities have not been rightly conceived by majority of the institutions or faculty members. In its true perspective extension education should not be viewed as a single subject but it is an amalgamation of sociology, journalism, psychology, economics besides our own disciplines like hygiene, nutrition, gynecology, medicine, LPM etc. and is the building blocks of its composite structure. Even the health services rendered at the doorsteps of livestock owners or out station services of any forms including breeding, feeding, management, preventive and health care practices are the primary component of extension services. In other words, **Extension education is an applied behavioral science, the knowledge of which is applied to bring about desirable changes in the behavioral complex of human beings usually through various strategies, program of change and by applying the latest scientific and technological innovations.**

10.2 Present status of Extension education at Veterinary Colleges / Universities / Extension centers

Department of Extension education is one of the mandatory requirements at Veterinary colleges as per the Minimum Standards of

Veterinary education, Regulations, 2008. Thus colleges have created the department but hardly any institution possess qualified faculty in veterinary & animal husbandry extension education. Majority of these faculty members drafted from other disciplines or with orientation in extension education from agricultural sciences are not expected to deliver to their fullest capacity. It is also largely true that the department is relatively poor in infrastructural facilities and the type of support needed to mange even the campus activities/ programs are not readily available.

Universities are the treasure of knowledge, new ideas, new techniques and new processes which could be effectively disseminated to the end users mainly the livestock farming community through the technical staff of the extension and associated departments. More often than not because of the lack of coordination and convergence, the much needed new knowledge, ideas, innovation, techniques, concepts and practices remain within the four walls of the university/colleges and do not reach the end users due to Lack of priority of the institutions, availability of less number of extension personal, insufficient resources and other commitment enforced on them. The universities/colleges are of course organizing farmer fairs, training, and workshops and using print and electronic media to reach the farmers. Some universities have developed help lines (24x7) for the farming community to reach subject matter specialists. Expert talks on Radio and TV channels are available in form of krishi darshans, pashupalan programs etc.

Regional research and training centers as well as KVK"s are mandated to perform extension activities, impart trainings and extend farm advisory services in their operational area. It is also a cause of concern that there are very few KVKs attached to veterinary universities. Further, in other KVKs which are mainly attached to SAUs normally, have hardly few scientists from livestock disciplines are attached. Even in State of Punjab about 50% KVK under SAU are running without any animal science specialist. The ICAR must review its existing policy and ensure proportionate share of KVKs for this sector.

The State governments should also strengthen its research cum training centers to effectively discharge responsibilities towards transfer of technological practices in livestock sector. It is heartening to note that the Rajasthan Government has sanctioned Veterinary University Training and Research Centre (VUTRC) under Directorate of Extension

RAJUVAS for each district of Rajasthan. Posts of training organizer (associate professor) and two training assistants (assistant professors) along with other supporting staff have been provided to effectively run these centre. The other states should also create similar centers to strengthen livestock extension programs.

A glaring picture has emerged through the National sample survey report of NSSO, that only 5% of the farmers' households in India have access to Animal Husbandry as against 40% on crop farming. Further, the fund allocation to this sector is hardly 1%. Such an abysmal picture should act as an eye opener for policy planners and plan executers. It calls for an emergent need to address such imbalances.

Another stressing point is that, there is a dire need to up-date the syllabus of both UG and PG courses to acquaint the students with practical problems existing in the field and the ways to tackles them through proper planning.

The broad objectives through which extension education/services should be planned and executes.

10.3 Objectives and Goals

- To uplift the livestock sector by educating the livestock farmers with latest and scientific practices on breeding, feeding, management and health aspects.
- To provide effective extension services in the field of animal husbandry and veterinary side.
- Promoting self employment opportunities to the rural masses including unemployed youth and rural woman in livestock farming.
- Motivation of rural masses to adopt livestock farming with recommended practices.
- Refining of indigenous practices for their easy adoption.

10.4 Constraints for Livestock Extension Services

In-fact extension education as well as its services in livestock sector is basically agriculture driven and as a practice efforts were / are being made to copy from agriculture extension programs and tried to transfix in veterinary sector. Though, the VCI for the first time enforced the creation of independent department of veterinary and animal husbandry Extension through the MSVE, Regulations 1993 and introduced 3 courses of 7 credit hours but the colleges/institutions were slow in understanding the relevance of this department and importance of this subject. To carry out the teaching requirements, these courses were allotted to teachers from allied sciences. In the process of revising MSVE, Regulations in 2008, attempts were made to make these courses more practical oriented but in true sense extension education failed to get its right place and space in curricular building of the graduate.

It is also a fact that very few colleges started offering PG education in extension, thereby resulting in less available expertise in extension. Unless a vigorous approach is adopted in producing human capital in the parent discipline of veterinary and animal husbandry extension education, real approach in transfer of technological practice would continue to remain a setback in near future also. A few of the serious constraints hampering transfer of technological practices are;

1. Remained under the domain of agriculture extension
2. Considering livestock farming as the subsidiary occupation.
3. Lack of trained manpower (in terms of livestock extension)
4. Lack of farmers friendly technologies.
5. Lack of communication between extension-farmers, scientist-extension worker, and inter-institutional level hampers the flow of required information to the end users.
6. Lack of resources per se at institutional and state level.
7. Less responsiveness of the livestock farmers
8. Lower user friendly credit facility
9. Poor availability of modern extension methods viz. information kiosks, e-extension, mobile extension units
10. Poor involvement of industries in Extension
11. Lack of proper marketing and pricing policies
12. Mindset of the veterinarians especially younger one to restrict to white collar job
13. Extensive working area (jurisdiction under his command) of a veterinarian due to less availability of competent human resource

10.5 What Livestock Farmers Need?

It has been a general practice that the input of the user agencies/ end users are rarely sought while formalization of the policies and programs. An attempt has been made to compile some of the basic needs of the farming community. This list can be further expanded in consultations with large group of livestock farmers.

1. Small dairy farmers – need survivability
2. Organized Market/ Mandi facility
3. MSP system of livestock produce
4. Feeding of balanced ration, mineral mixture
5. Improved fodder production
6. Modern shed construction
7. Health control and production improving measures.
8. Easy and long term credit facility
9. Specialized door step extension services or paid extension services
10. Livestock farming at par with agriculture or industry in term of government support
11. Hi-tech consultancy for progressive dairy farmers
12. 24X7 hrs technical input services

10.6 Approach for Strengthening Livestock Extension

Some premise need to be stated from the onset:

- Development of new livestock extension system rather than agriculture based
- Relying more on ICT (Information, communication and technology) is the need of the hour. Like in Pondicherry and Tamil Nadu "e-Kiosk" and "Livestock Guru" type program need to be replicated in other states in vernacular language.
- Mobile network service can be included in this e-extension services as it is now a basic need and every farmer have it. Providing timely information, forecasting, flash information can be spread in no time to masses via mobile. Whatsapp type application (AHapp and LHaap) can be made available for download from

institute website which provides basic information. Specialist's service can be sought thereafter as and when needed.

- Availability of video films on different aspects of livestock farming and success stories of proven and progressive farmers.
- Establishing the connecting link with the line departments for similar type of knowledge transfer otherwise two types of information on single topic often perplex the farmers which results in reluctance to adopt technology. Message should be simple, clear and uniform
- Area and need based approach should be adopted for effective adaptation of the technologies.
- **"We are for the farmers, farmers are not for us"** So, language should not be a bar between scientist and farmers. Every extension worker must be well acquainted with the local terminologies used by rural people. The right step is to teach them these terminologies at under graduation level.
- Farmer led extension approach should be undertaken for horizontal and vertical learning.
- Livestock Extension Bank or Fodder and Feed Formulation Banks for tackling nutritional aspects are required to be developed.
- Rationale use of available resources or alternate sources should be sought to strengthen the extension activities
- Whatever strategies are adopted, regardless of the approach or system used, they must be suited to local conditions; flexible enough to be able to respond to changing circumstances;
- Gender based approach need to be promoted especially in area where orthodox practices are still prevailing. Women have a prominent role in small-scale animal production systems, but, in many places it is difficult to deal directly with female household members for obvious reasons. Female extension scientist should be encouraged to provide them doorstep training or other inputs.
- Feasibilities should be explored to declare World Animal Welfare Day or Healthy Animal Day etc.

10.7 To achieve this, the present set up needs through overhauling by providing the need based and door step extension services by the following ways

- Foremost step is strengthening of existing extension wing in terms of man power and infrastructure.
- UG and PG curriculum should be redesigned to make the student well versed with extension methodologies for effective dissemination of technologies/services.
- Successful models of extension developed by ICAR institutes & veterinary universities needs to be adopted/ replicated.
- Veterinarians need to be trained in extension delivery system and para vet should also be trained for livestock technologies for wider coverage.
- Every newly recruited faculty member of the veterinary institute should undertake training in extension so that he is sensitized and well versed with extension and rural people, accordingly his mind set will automatically be tilted towards the practical aspect.
- Separate cadre and position for undertaking livestock extension at block, district and state level and suitable people recruited.
- Public private Partnership should be promoted to cover the every nook and corner
- Dedicated regional research and training centre (RRTC), PashuVigyan Kendra/Pashu Palak Help Centre/Pashu Palan Information Centres should be established at different places to cater the need of masses.
- OFT (on farm trial) and OFD (on farm demonstration) should be given more weightage as seeing and doing has more pronounced affect than listening.
- Reorientation of grass root field functionaries for extension education and services.
- Veterinary polytechnic, Polyclinic and public Animal Farms can be developed as the extension cum demonstration unit to strengthen the extension services.
- Farmer's field school, women self-help groups, NGO's can be integrated to impart the training especially for women farmers at field level.

10.8 Agencies Associated for Livestock Extension

The following figure depicids the agencies associated with livestock extension.

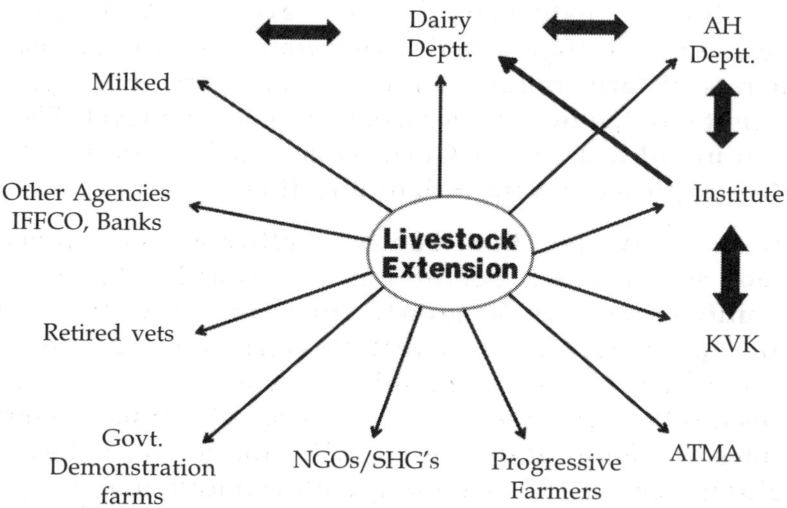

AGENCIES FOR LIVESTOCK EXTENSION

10.9 The following figure present proposed model for extension wing at the State Level

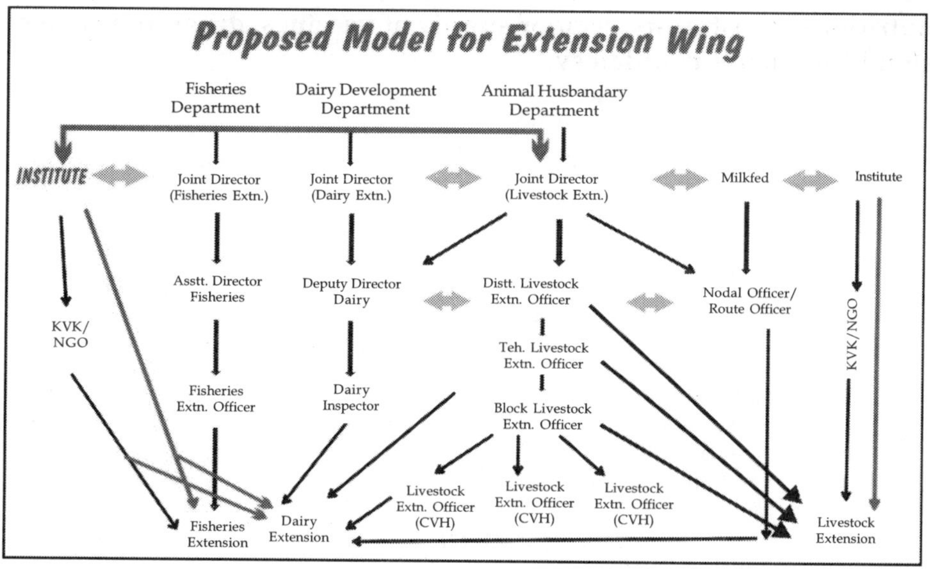

10.10 Epilogue

Beside the above mentioned suggestion/steps for strengthening of extension education at varsity/college level, the Govt. may also restructured/reframe its existing sources to make the extension more effective. Animal husbandry, dairy department, NGO, private industries, animal welfare societies, cooperative societies, gaushala, and progressive farmers can be interwoven under public private partnership to do the needed extension at grass root level. Though it seem an uphill task, but if Govt. wills, it will be definitely an affirmative approach toward a right direction.

Now, it is very vivid that country's' cultivable land cannot be increased, so livestock sector has to shoulder the greater responsibility to improve the growth rate of the agriculture sector. So, seeing the importance of livestock extension education and services, conducive policies should be framed at National level, which ensures the strengthening of infrastructure, human resource at institutes as well as at outstation, KVK and Regional Research and Training centers (RRTC) along with committed and regular grants for these. The provision of first aid, disease diagnosis, feed, fodder and milk testing, skill developments, project preparation, knowledge/information sharing may be facilitated at these regional stations to provide composite services and training at the center.

For enhancing and sustaining productivity, commercialization of livestock production, overcoming of animal diseases and nutritional constraints, regular supply of vaccines, drugs and semen should be made mandatory.

❑❑❑

Chapter-11

An Ideal Teaching Veterinary Clinical Complex (TVCC)

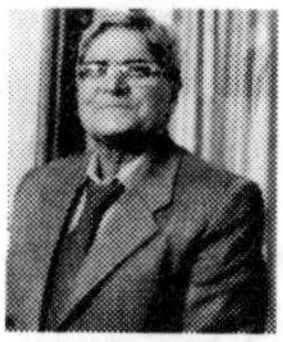

JIT SINGH, MVSc, Ph.D, FISVS, FNAVS
Former Professor and Head
Department of Surgery and Radiology,
College of Veterinary and Animal Sciences,
LUVAS Hisar and Dean, College of Veterinary & Animal Sciences,
Navania, (RAJUVAS) Udaipur

Veterinary Science, unlike human medical science, is a complex and diversified discipline as it deals with number of species with widely different anatomical and physiological differences and wide variations in mechanism of diseases, methods of diagnosis and response to drugs/medicines. Therefore, a clinic also requires species Specific facilities. Moreover, in India there are diverse agro climatic zones and domestication of different species as a majority may also differ. Thus it may not be possible to bench-mark one plan of a teaching veterinary clinical complex and every clinic plan may have to be adjusted/modified according to local needs but by including minimum essential requirements for other species too so that training process encompasses all.

A Teaching Veterinary hospital is a hospital which provides clinical education and training to future and current veterinarians and para-veterinary staff in addition to providing diagnostic and treatment facilities to deliver medical care to the animal patients. In India teaching veterinary hospitals are a part of veterinary colleges only and independent teaching hospitals of wider regional or national animal health system do not exist so far.

Aims and objective of an ideal Teaching Veterinary hospital

Basically the aim of a teaching hospital is to provide basic training in diagnosis and treatment of animal patients as a hands-on training schedule and to provide comprehensive training to interns and post-graduate students of clinical disciplines. However a clinical hospital is a very good resource of research material too for faculty as well as post - graduate students. As per Veterinary council of India MSVE regulations-2008, in teaching hospital animal patient information should be utilized to the maximum while observing principles of animal welfare and ethics. In case of cases of academic interest or typical cases of teaching value free maintenance should be provided for the benefit of Students.

In case of death/euthanasia detailed necropsy be demonstrated and specimens should be preserved. In addition clinical conferences should be arranged on typical cases where both faculty and interns should be in attendance. There is no need to stress that services in a teaching hospitals should be available round the clock.

As has already been stated an ideal teaching hospital should have core business of clinical services, teaching and also research. Therefore, aims and objectives should also be framed accordingly. Following are some points:

1. Clinical services

a) To provide efficient and effective services

b) To be the major specialist services provider for the target animal population.

c) To provide additional services such as ambulatory services and in form of clinical camps.

d) To help Govt. veterinary services in vaccination programmes and other preventive measures.

2. Research and Development

To use patient information and clinical material for research purposes all the time keeping in mind animal welfare principles and well being of patient and benefit of owner.

3. Teaching and Learning

a) To ensure that staff provides safe, effective and quality patient care.

b) To encourage culture of innovation.

c) To provide effective client counseling wherever required.

d) To ensure that each typical case becomes a source of knowledge for faculty and trainees without jeopardizing the interest of patient and client.

e) To inculcate in trainees personal commitment to the profession as per veterinarians oath.

Basic Infrastructure

As has already been stated infrastructure has to be adjusted as per local needs, however, basic structure is being spelled out common for all species and special requirements for different species are listed at the end. One major requirement is that building structure should be well ventilated and eco-friendly and provisions made keeping in view the climate.

1. General routine health care

Facilities in form of space, furniture etc. and equipments should be created for physical examination, vaccinations and to treat minor illness by interns under supervision of faculty.

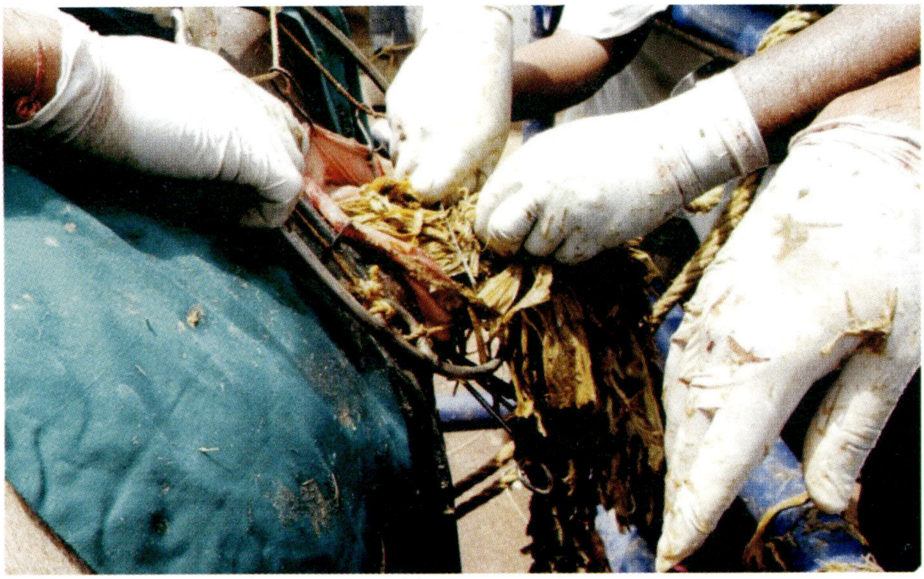

Rumentomy, TVCC GADVASU

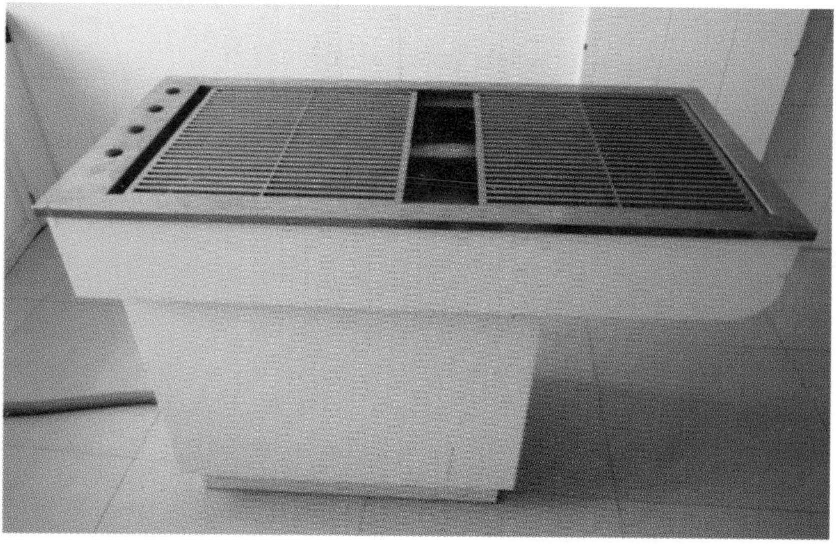

Scrub Table (Designed at TVCC, Palampur)

2. Special Services

Veterinary Science has made tremendous progress in diagnostics and therapeutic measures. Therefore, the areas which require special services are listed below :

a) Anaesthesia and pain management.
b) Emergency critical care.
c) Imaging techniques e.g. radiography, ultrasound etc.
d) Well equipped diagnostic laboratory using state of the art techniques.
e) Dentistry.
f) Dermatology.
g) Trauma centre to handle accidental cases including neurology to diagnose and treat spiral cord, nerves and muscle abnormality.
h) Physiotherapy
i) Internal medicine
j) Soft tissue surgery for abdomen and thorax including laparoscopic and thoracoscopic techniques.
k) Ophthalmology.
l) Orthopaedic surgery.

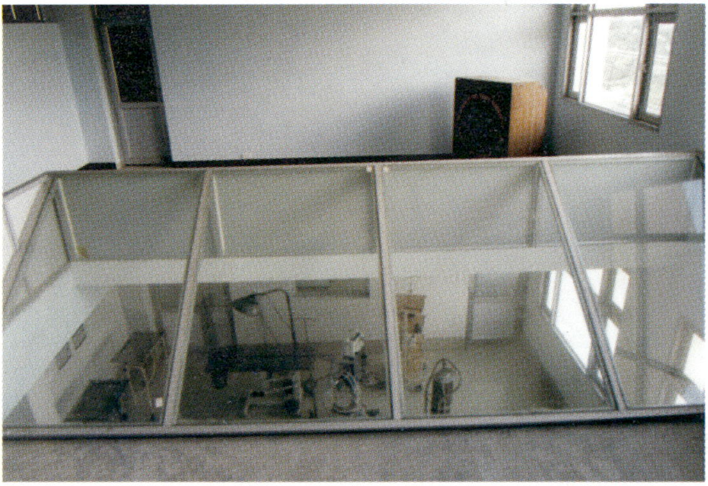

Instructional Surgery Operation Theater, TVCC Palampur

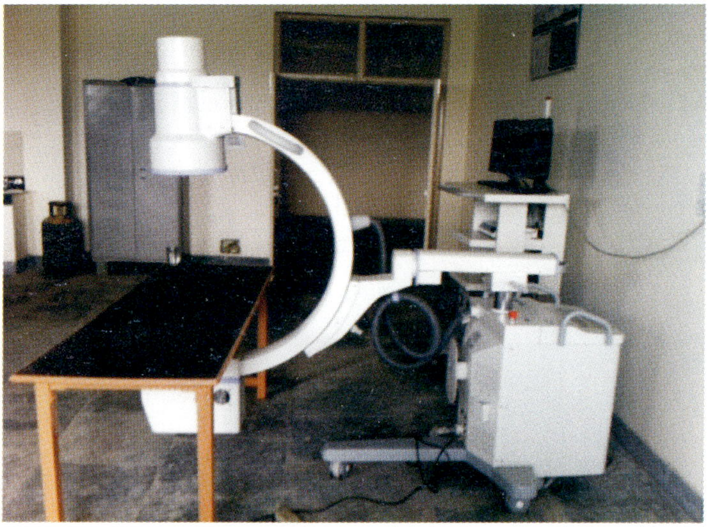

C-ARM, KCVAS Amritsar

Additional requirements are

Pet Animals

1. Diagnosis and treatment of behavior problems through modifications and medications.
2. Cardiology.
3. Pet animals also require comfortable kennels with provision of temperature control.

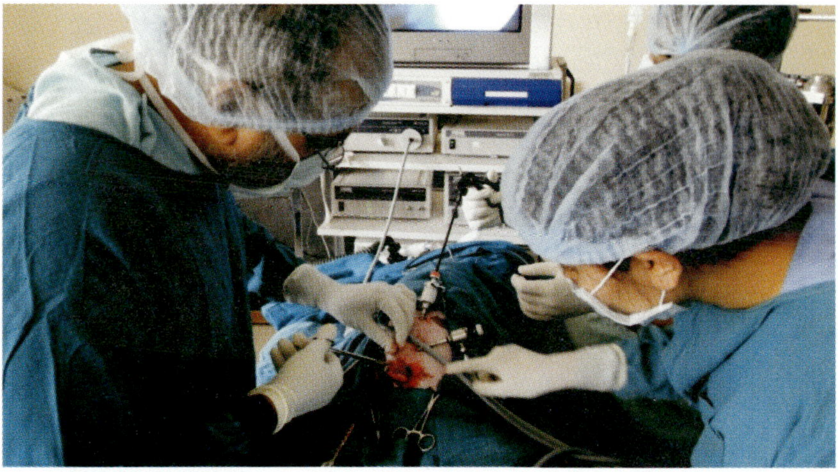

Endoscopic Surgery for colic in Horses, TVCC GADVASU

Equines

Where equine patients are good in number services of a Ferrier should be available. Recovery room's floor and walls require padding to avoid injury during recovery from anaesthesia. Stalls should be well ventilated with comfortable bedding and floor. For standing procedures the chute should be specially designed. Similarly operation tables should be specially designed so that animal can be easily restrained while in standing position itself and then table can be tilted back.

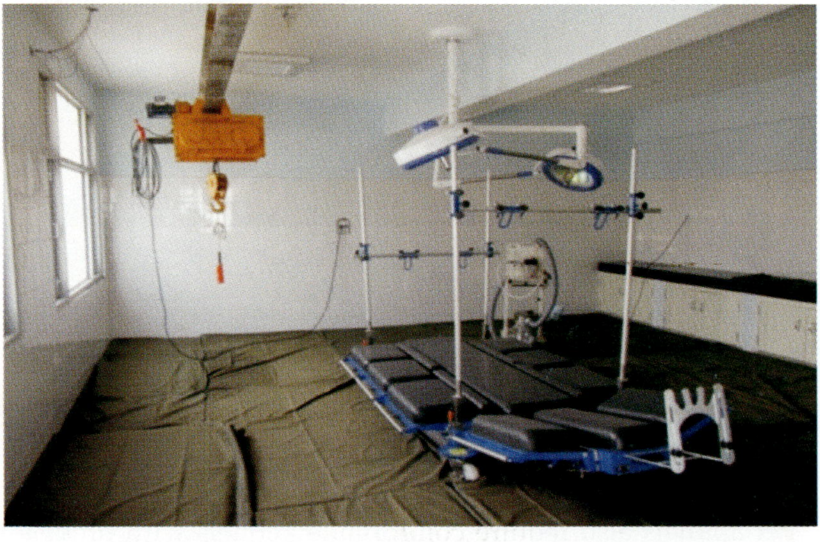

Equine Surgical Operation Theater, TVCC Palampur

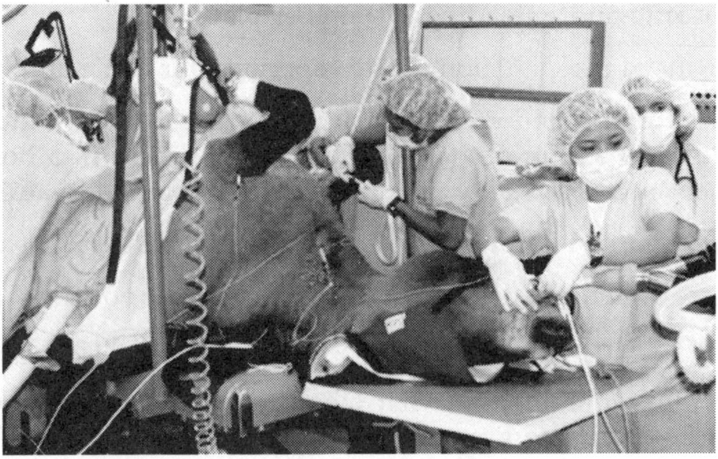

Vasectomy in a Horse, TVCC GADVASU

Other large and small animals

Restraining chutes should be comfortable and designed as per height of the animal. For calves, sheep & goats specially designed chutes are available. Ruminants are prone to slip and so flooring should be antislippery.

For Birds

Special wards should be there for different species so that mixture of species is not there. Wards must be provided with temperature control system. Desert coolers can be used for summers provided humidity is not high. During winter filament oil heaters should be used instead of room heaters to avoid direct heating so that walls become warm and temperature can be controlled according to requirements.

Basic Other Requirements

1. There should be efficient bio-security system to prevent hospital infections transmission to patients.
2. Special facilities for patients with contagious diseases (isolation wards).
3. Facilities to handle recumbent animals, both for small and large animal.
4. Ambulatory services along with animal transport facilities.

5. Loading and unloading systems or platform.
6. Artificial insemination centre especially for cattle and buffalo.
7. Comfortable indoor wards. It should be kept in mind that in India owners prefer to stay near their animals in a hospital so client accommodation should be near the indoor wards.
8. Post-mortem hall with carcase lifting and disposal system.
9. Arrangements for biomedical waste disposal as per law requirements.

Needless to emphasize that what has been written here is as a basic and special requirements, and manpower, space, equipments etc. would be required to complete the picture. It is not feasible to list all these here and much will depend upon local needs too.

Some floor plan models for canine and pet centers animal hospitals are depicted below :

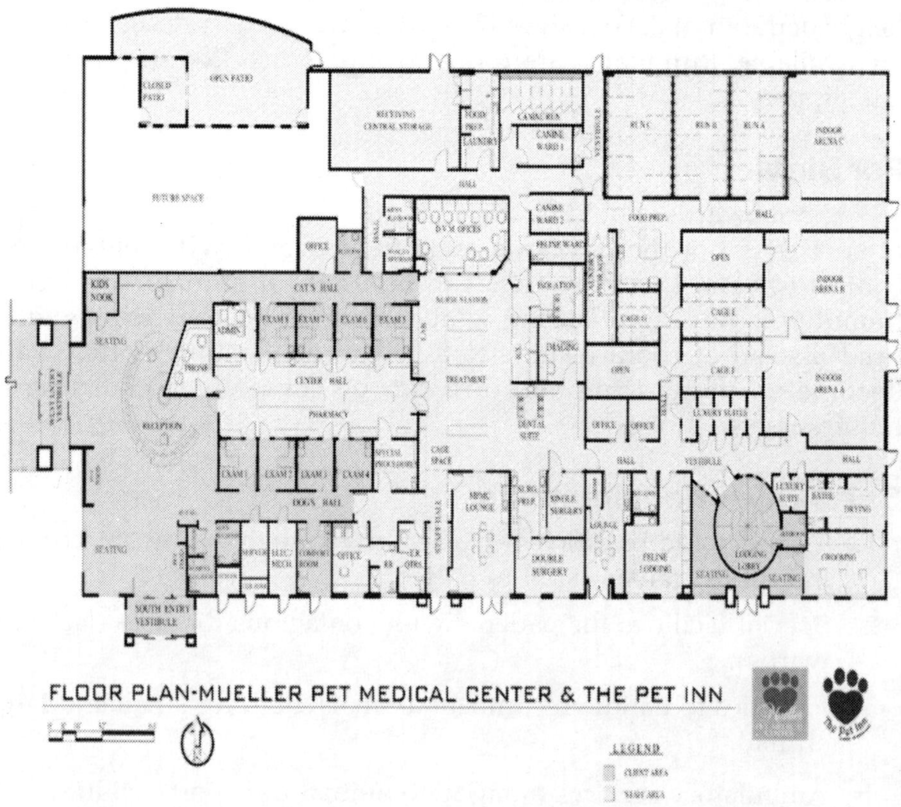

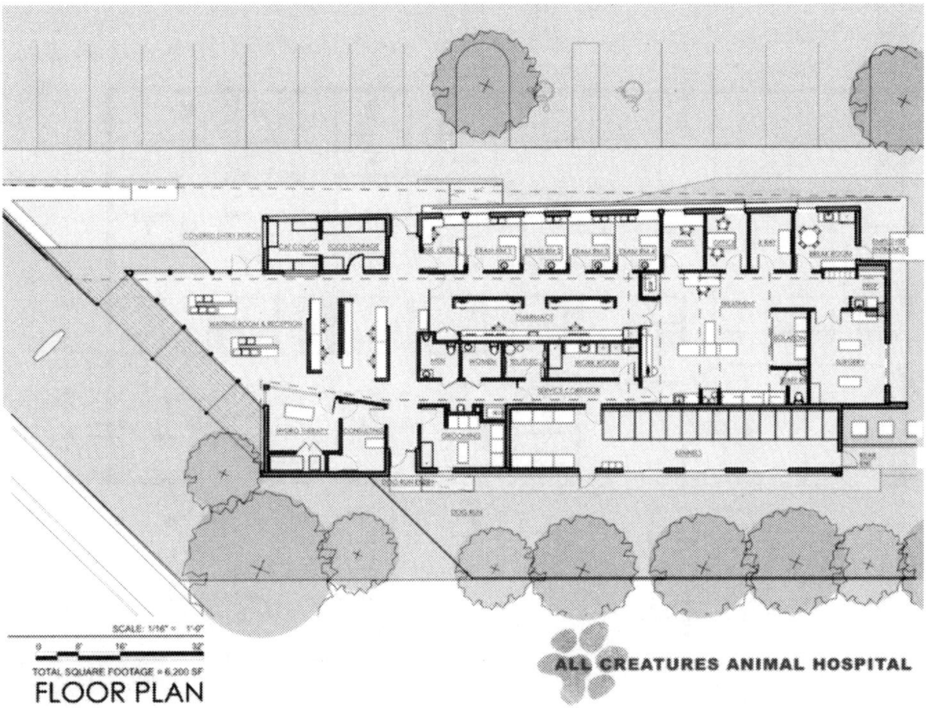
SCALE: 1/16" = 1'-0"
TOTAL SQUARE FOOTAGE = 6,200 SF
FLOOR PLAN
ALL CREATURES ANIMAL HOSPITAL

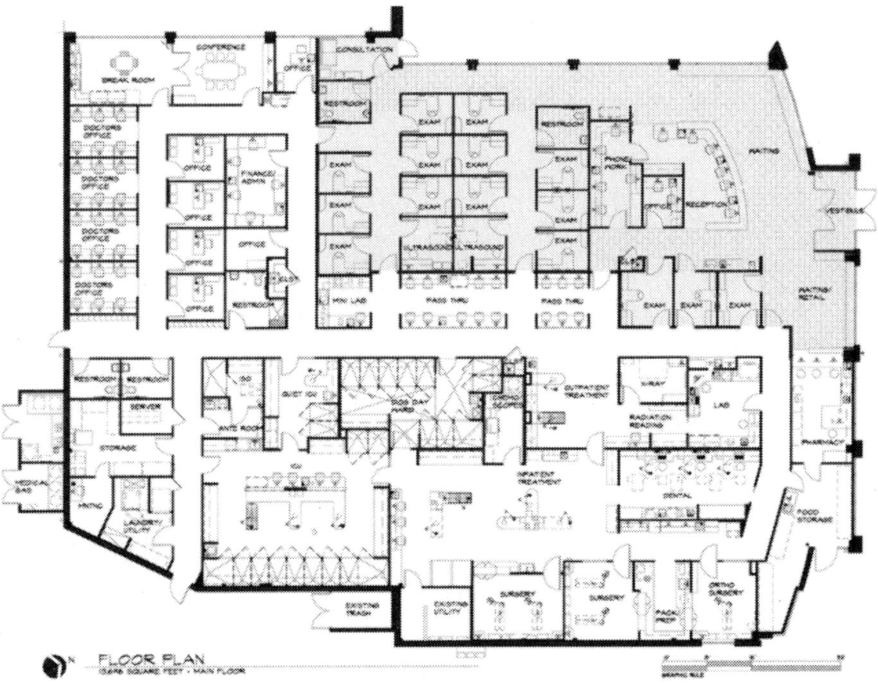
FLOOR PLAN

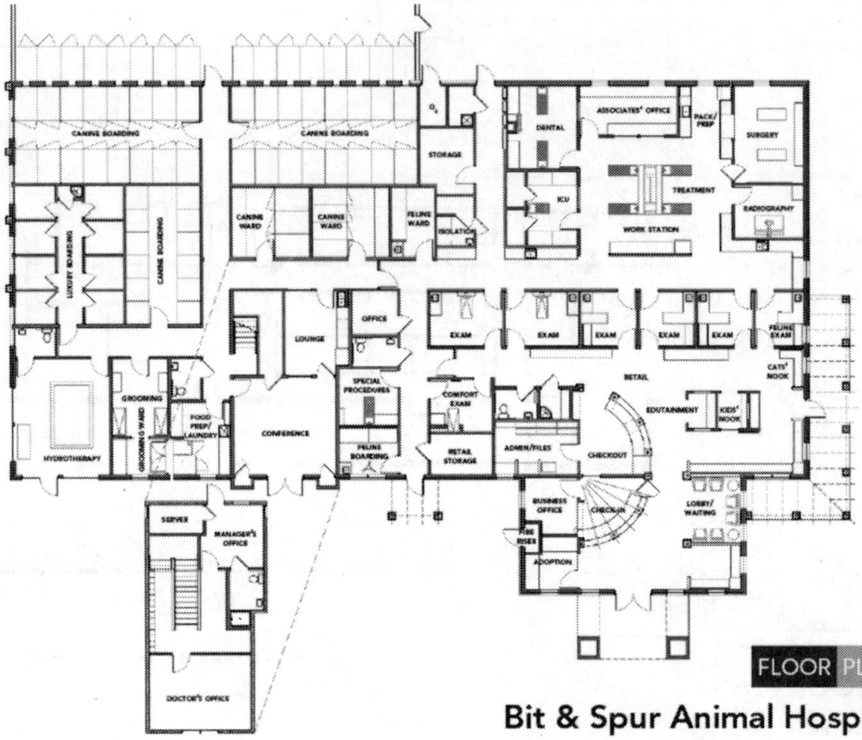

FLOOR PLAN

Bit & Spur Animal Hospital

Chapter-12

Need to Strengthen Clinical Diagnosis in Animal Health Management

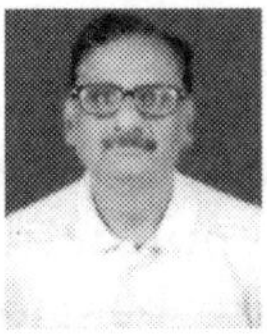 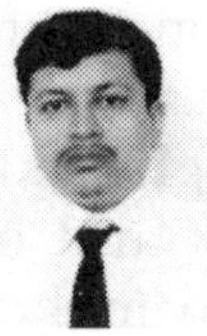

Dr. A.K.SRIVASTAVA & Dr. MANOJ KUMAR*
Professor and Head and Assistant Professor*
Khalsa College of Veterinary and Animal Sciences, Amritsar 143002

'More mistakes are made by not looking than by not knowing' – Anonymous

12.1 Introduction

Clinical examination is a fundamental part of the process of veterinary diagnosis. It provides the veterinarian with the information essential for determining the disease (s) producing the clinical abnormalities. Additionally, the information obtained from the detailed clinical examination assists the veterinarian in determining the severity of the patho-physiological alterations present in the body. Without a proficient clinical examination it is almost impossible to arrive at an accurate diagnosis so as not to devise appropriate treatment and control measures.

The importance of laboratory diagnosis has increased manifolds during last couple of the years due to emergence and re-emergence of various infectious and contagious diseases in animals. The occurrence of new diseases in animals and poultry also created havoc in the society, particularly of those having zoonotic importance. The outbreak of avian influenza, swine influenza, Japanese encephalitis, leptospirosis and glanders in different states of India for last couple of years caused concern not only to the veterinarian and medicos but the entire administration and economic machinery of the country, resulting in establishment of Bio safety level 3 and 4 laboratories in the country for the microbial isolation and disease diagnosis.

The foremost motive of a practicing veterinarian is providing the most economical method of diagnosis and treatment of sick and injured animals. This objective is more relevant to the veterinarian engaged in farm animal practices and has to cope with cost constraints in everyday practices.

The diagnosis, treatment and control of diseases of farm animals rely heavily on the history provided by the owner, results of the clinical examination of animals on the farm and the careful examination of the environment and managemental techniques. This requires the veterinarian to become highly skilled in obtaining relevant and useful history on the first visit and in conducting an adequate clinical examination in order to make the best diagnosis possible, and economically so that the treatment and control measures can be instituted as soon as possible. On the farmer's doorstep, a veterinarian will not have access to a microbiological facility to determine whether the acutely pneumonic buffalo is suffering from pneumonic pasteurellosis or not. The practitioner must become a proficient diagnostician and a skilful user of the physical diagnostic skills of visual observation, auscultation, palpation, percussion, succession, ballottement and olfactory perceptions.

Improving the clinical diagnostic skills of veterinary graduates and practitioners is of utmost importance especially for the owner of livestock mostly having low per capita income in India. It is not a hidden fact that most government veterinary hospitals have poor infrastructures and in such a setting it is almost impossible for the veterinarian to rely on clinical and laboratory diagnostic equipment to arrive at a proper diagnosis.

It is also important to appreciate that most of the veterinary teaching hospitals and referral hospitals have sophisticated imaging and clinical pathology equipments due to better funding and regulatory requirements. For the purpose of animal disease diagnosis, Government of India and the State Government have set up a chain of diagnostic laboratories in the country.

Central Disease Diagnostic Laboratory
CADRAD, IVRI, Izatnagar

↓

Regional Disease Diagnostic Laboratories

↓

NERDDL Guwahati	ERDDL Kolkata	WRDDL Pune	NRDDL Jalandhar	SRDDL Bangalore
1. Assam	1. West Bengal	1. Maharashtra	1. Jammu & Kashmir	1. Karnataka
2. Sikkim	2. Bihar	2. Gujarat	2. Punjab	2. Andhra Pradesh
3. Arunachal Pradesh	3. Orissa	3. Madhya Pradesh	3. Haryana	3. Tamilnadu
4. Manipur	4. Jharkhand	4. Chattisgarh	4. Himachal Pradesh	4. Kerala
5. Meghalaya	5. Andaman & Nicobar Island	5. Goa	5. Rajasthan	5. Pondicherry
6. Nagaland		6. Daman & Due	6. Chandigarh	
			7. Delhi	

Establishment of a few regional disease diagnostic labs in different states of India is an iota in the vast field of disease diagnosis in view of the huge population of the livestock prevailing in the country. However, these diagnostic laboratories dealing with clinical specimens also requires ISO 17025 certification while non-clinical testing laboratories require good laboratory practices (GLP) certification.

Clinical teaching faculty and veterinary practitioners are used to the assistance provided by such diagnostic modalities. However, the transition of the student from an academic setting to stand alone clinical practice puts him in a state of apprehension. A practitioner who is well equipped in the clinical diagnostic skills finds himself in good stead and is more willing and ready to serve the rural poor.

12.2 Constraints in Imparting Effective Clinical Skills to Veterinary Students and Possible Remedial Measures

12.2.1 Lack of sufficient clinical faculty

Currently this is the most important problem encountered by most of the veterinary teaching institutions of our country and with no short term solution in sight. The situation prevails despite availability of large number of veterinarians who have post graduate qualifications and are very much interested in an academic career.

Also, the regulatory requirement for faculty strength in clinical disciplines is similar to other disciplines despite the fact that clinical skills cannot be imparted in the way a 'normal' practical class is conducted. This becomes very much apparent if we analyze the staffing pattern of those veterinary teaching institutions of the country that have a reputation of imparting better clinical training.

12.2.2 Lack of career incentives for clinical teaching staff

Effective clinical teaching in veterinary teaching institutions requires motivated and enthusiastic clinical teachers. However, in general, the career prospects for academics (including clinical faculty) working in university environments remains firmly linked to the blue sky research and more so on research publication in high impact peer reviewed journals.

Although it is important to create a positive research environment, it is equally important that veterinary teaching institutions understand the societal need for the optimally trained veterinary clinician and that they do not adapt a simplistic 'one size fits all' strategy for career bench marks. It is important to encourage those academics with particular skills and interest to pursue clinical, teaching or professional development tracks.

To improve teaching and training environment it is necessary to incentivize activities which are student and society centered and not solely career centered.

12.3 Poorly Structured Curriculum and Pedagogy

12.3.1 Less than desired clinical orientation of basic, preclinical and paraclinical subjects and faculty

When the current curriculum and teaching methods of basic and preclinical subjects are put in sight, it becomes obvious that they are taught in isolation to real life clinical conditions. Practical syllabi and teaching style of most of these subjects is too much laboratory oriented. It has been a personal experience that most of the basic and preclinical faculty tends to maintain a 'safe distance' from teaching hospital and diseased animals for the purpose of teaching. It feels appalling when final year student who have already gone through all the basic and preclinical courses fluently narrates ethio-pathogenesis, epidemiology, clinical signs, clinical pathology etc. of canine distemper and says he/she has never seen a single 'dancing dog' in his/her life. It is beyond comprehension that how applied anatomy or systemic pathology or clinical biochemistry etc. could be taught effectively to students without exposing them to clinical cases.

Even before the onset of the formal stages of hands-on clinical education, the teaching hospital is a fantastic teaching resource in the pre-clinical years. Every case offers a learning opportunity. Clinical pathology instruction based on actual clinical cases seen in the teaching hospital is much more likely to catch the intense interest of pre-clinical students than would other ways of teaching clinical pathology. Reorienting the curriculum and teaching methodology of basic and preclinical subjects would definitely help students to integrate their theoretical knowledge with the real life problems.

The following quote of the famous physician -Sir William Osler sums it all.

"To study the phenomena of disease without books is to sail an uncharted sea, while to study books without patients is not to go to sea at all".

12.3.2 Didactic theoretical teaching instead of case based learning and discussions

Teachings of clinical subjects also suffer from similar deficiencies as discussed previously for basic and pre clinical subjects. i.e. overemphasis on theoretical lecturing instead of arming the students with essential skills required for diagnosis and management of clinical cases. While teaching clinical subjects, students will tremendously be benefitted from clinical case based discussions. This necessitates effective management of clinical case records.

12.3.3 Over burdened curriculum and too frequent curriculum changes

The present curriculum of Veterinary Council of India has put tremendous load not only on the subject matters but various extracurricular activities in the form of essential non credit courses. This has indeed over burdened the undergraduates who try to find narrow gaps in the process of elaborate clinical practices that also includes veterinary laboratory diagnosis.

12.4 Insufficient Case Load

There is rarely a place on earth which is not inhabited by humans and animals or where animals do not fall sick. Therefore, insufficient case load at a teaching hospital only reflect the type of service being provided by the hospital to the society. However, one thing that is often observed is the species variation in cases presented to the hospital. Veterinary colleges or hospitals located in or near to metropolises receive more cases of companion animals and those located in smaller towns receive more cases of farm animals.

In any case, low case load necessitates efficient utilization of cases presented in the form of teaching material without jeopardizing the best interest of the patient. This may include video-graphy of the clinical picture, any procedure/ surgery performed and preservation of case record with all the clinical pathology findings for future reference.

Real size simulators such as 'colic horse' and 'dystocia cow' have also been developed and can be used to simulate clinical scenario. A lot of good and free videos are available online e.g. on YouTube which can be used to demonstrate various clinical procedures to the students.

12.5 Submission of Poor Clinical Samples to Laboratory

For the accurate and quick diagnosis, the clinical materials must be submitted scientifically and in accordance with the standard protocols. The various types of samples that includes biological fluids and morbid material viz. blood as whole in anticoagulants, serum, blood smears, urine, milk, CSF, effusion fluid, semen, synovial fluid, aspirated materials form natural orifices, rectal washing, impression smears, scraping smears, biopsy materials, fecal materials and post mortem materials. There appears practical difficulty in using the low quality clinical materials for diagnosis because of improper collection and preservation. The quantity of the submitted specimens may also matters in the process of diagnosis. The veterinary institutions across the country has developed the veterinary polytechnic for diploma courses like Live Stock Extension Officer (LEO), Veterinary Compounder, Veterinary nurse, Pharmacy etc. to train the para-clinical staff to perform their duties successfully in the hospitals and in the field.

12.6 Poor Communication and Interpersonal Skills in the Students

The ultimate goal of veterinary professional education is to prepare students for the versatile role one has to play in the society; and to effectively play that role one must have excellent communication and interpersonal skills. Good communication skill is not limited to linguistic proficiency alone.

Successful clinical diagnosis in veterinary practice relies heavily on the history provided by the client or to be precise, on the tact and communication proficiency of the veterinarian in obtaining as much useful information as possible. A practicing clinician often finds himself playing the role of a psychoanalyst, trying to extract relevant information from the client and trying to always empathize with the client even when sometimes he does not want to. There are several published reports which indicate that foremost cause of professional failure of practicing veterinarians is not the lack of technical skills but poor communication skills. In veterinary practices, non-compliance of veterinarian's instructions is one of the most important causes of treatment failure which ultimately leads to client dissatisfaction. Poor communication on part of the veterinarian is often the primary cause of the misunderstanding.

Introduction of course titled 'Veterinarians in Society' in the BVSc & AH curriculum in the recent curriculum change by VCI is a move in the right direction. All that is needed is to encourage students to interact with livestock and pet owners in a meaningful and purposeful manner, first under supervision and then on their own.

12.7 Non Practicing of Routine Clinical Conference

The common endemic diseases are easily diagnosed by the practitioners with satisfactory remedial measures for treating the disease. In the present time, the pathogens have changed their molecular configuration so as to become superbug (antibiotic resistant) or changed the pattern of manifestations of disease. Under these circumstances, it has presented a great challenge to the clinician for their diagnosis and the proper remedial measures.

To cope up these hard tasks, specialization and super specialization has widely emerged in various branches of science which symbolizes the advancement in the diagnosis and treatment of the various invasive and noninvasive diseases. The referral hospital needs to have the trained and experienced human resources so that the referred cases from the village and district levels of hospitals may be diagnosed and properly treated. There is need to have the various specialized persons to handle the difficult and obstinate cases. In this matter, a clinical conference comprised of the experts of clinical and paraclinical subjects may be organized routinely to arrive at the conclusive diagnosis. The expert of clinical subjects that includes the Medicine, Surgery and Gynecology and paraclinical subjects like Pathology, Microbiology, and

Biochemistry etc. may be invited to participate in the conference as a routine practice. If it is institutional referral Teaching Veterinary Clinical Complex (TVCC), the students of 4th & 5th years and internship students may also join to impart clinical knowledge and for better understanding of the disease. The outcome of the conference may suggest the use of certain routine diagnostic tests or advanced diagnostic tests and interpret the clinical laboratory results in order to arrive at the diagnosis of disease.

12.8 References

Jane R. Shaw. (2006). Four Core Communication Skills of Highly Effective Practitioners. Vet Clin Small Anim 36 385–396.

A.D.C. Jaarsma, D.H.J.M. Dolmans, A.J.J.A. Scherpbier and P. Van Beukelen.(2009) Educational approaches aimed at preparing students for professional veterinary practice. *Rev. sci. tech. Off. int. Epiz.*, 28 (2), 823-830.

Michael L. Doherty. (2012). 21st Century education in bovine health management: addressing the challenges. Proceedings of the 27th congress of the world association for buiatrics - Lisbon, Portugal, 31 - 35.

Smith, BP and Walsh, DA (2003). Teaching the art of clinical practice: the veterinary medical teaching hospital, private practice, and other externships. Journal of veterinary medical education, 30(3): 227 - 30.

Radostits, OM, Gay CC, Hinchkliff KW and Constable PD (2007). In: VETERINARY MEDICINE - A textbook of the diseases of cattle, horses, sheep, pigs and goats. Saunders, USA.

❑❑❑

Chapter-13

Diagnostic Imaging in Veterinary Practice

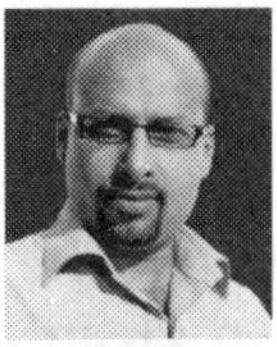

Dr. ADARSH KUMAR

Associate Professor, Department of Surgery and Radiology, Dr GC Negi College of Veterinary and Animal Sciences, CSK Himachal Pradesh KrishiVishvavidyalaya, Palampur (H.P.) Email: adarsh9kan@gmail.com

The art and science of Diagnostic Imaging became an integral part of veterinary health management through clinical and surgical interventions shortly after the exposure of the first radiographic films. The computer's ability to manipulate data has been applied to various imaging technologies, resulting in new images such as those seen with digital subtraction fluoroscopy, computed tomography (CT), magnetic resonance imaging (MRI), nuclear scintigraphy, and diagnostic ultrasono-graphy. These technological explosions have called for an expansion of veterinary expertise beyond traditional diagnostic radiology to include all types of diagnostic imaging. Of these newer technologies, ultrasono-graphy has gained popularity most rapidly among both veterinary specialists and small animal practitioners.

Diagnostic imaging has always been a mainstay of the **armamentarium** for the veterinarian. Veterinarians have limited resources available as regards history and routine screening procedures. Therefore, diagnostic imaging has a major role in the workup of numerous veterinary patients. An overreliance on diagnostic imaging has been observed by numerous clinicians; however, the move toward less invasive diagnostic procedures with a high precision of diagnosis has continued to drive this phenomenon.

Diagnostic radiology was utilized in for almost all livestock species and companion animals at all the veterinary institutions and in advanced states owned or in privately managed multi-facilities hospitals/poly-clinics in India. The use of diagnostic radiology expanded with improved knowledge, especially with better understanding of its diagnosis of various pathologic conditions. The use of diagnostic radiology abated somewhat with the advance of diagnostic ultrasonography; however, it has remained most acceptable diagnostic imaging in the veterinary profession. Presently, there is a major push to move from conventional analog film screen technology to computed and/or digital radiography. It is presumed that veterinary radiology will continue to follow the progression realized in human radiology.

Imaging plays a vital role in the evaluation of a sick patient. First and foremost images are a data set. The information is there. The clever and methodical evaluator can glean a vast amount of information from images. Integration into the work up of the patient requires insight and an abundance of skill and experience. Perseverance and dedication have no equal for the acquisition of a suitable skill set.

Historically, radiology has been confined to disease diagnosis, but the advent of interventional radiology brings exciting in roads into therapeutic techniques. Some alternative imaging techniques are indicated to narrow down the differential list and to plan a therapeutic approach. A range of imaging options is now available to veterinarians, including radiography (traditional and digital x-rays), fluoroscopy, ultransono-graphy, video endoscopy, lapararoscopy, nuclear scintigraphy (bone scan), computer-aided tomography (CT scan), and magnetic resonance imaging (MRI).

Radiography has long been a staple in imaging diagnostics for in clinics. They can be used to diagnose a variety of conditions, such as fractures, abscesses, malformations, abdominal and thoracic affections and lesions. With digital radiography, practitioners have immediate internal visualizations. Digital radiography today offers high-detail images that can be viewed on a computer screen for analysis, transferred to a radiographic monitor for evaluation and diagnosis, saved to a computer, saved to a disk, or e-mailed to another practitioner for a second opinion. Much like the individual digital cameras widely used today, the benefits of instant images and the ability to retake images to get a better shot are quite remarkable. The benefit to the patient is significant, because the diagnosis can be done on-site and treatment can commence immediately.

Another technology using X-rays is the fluoroscope. A **fluoroscope** is a real-time radiographic unit that has a flexible arm. The arm receives the X-rays and connects to a processor with a screen to display the image. It is portable and is used for procedures such as following a needle during joint injection and during surgery to ensure correct placement of implants. The image it produces is real-time imaging and its portability makes it a valuable tool for assisting with procedures.

Ultrasono-graphy uses sound waves to produce an image for diagnostic evaluation. The images are formed based upon the varying densities of soft tissue, organs, and bones. There are excellent portable units for use in the field that are used frequently in reproduction medicine to determine pregnancy, reproductive tract fitness, and fetal development. Many clinics have more powerful ultrasound units that can scan deep-tissue areas and also offer finer detail for assessing inured areas, abscesses, etc. Ultrasound can be used for assessing the abdominal areas and organs, cardiac evaluation, lung and respiratory tract evaluation, tendon and ligament studies, and more.

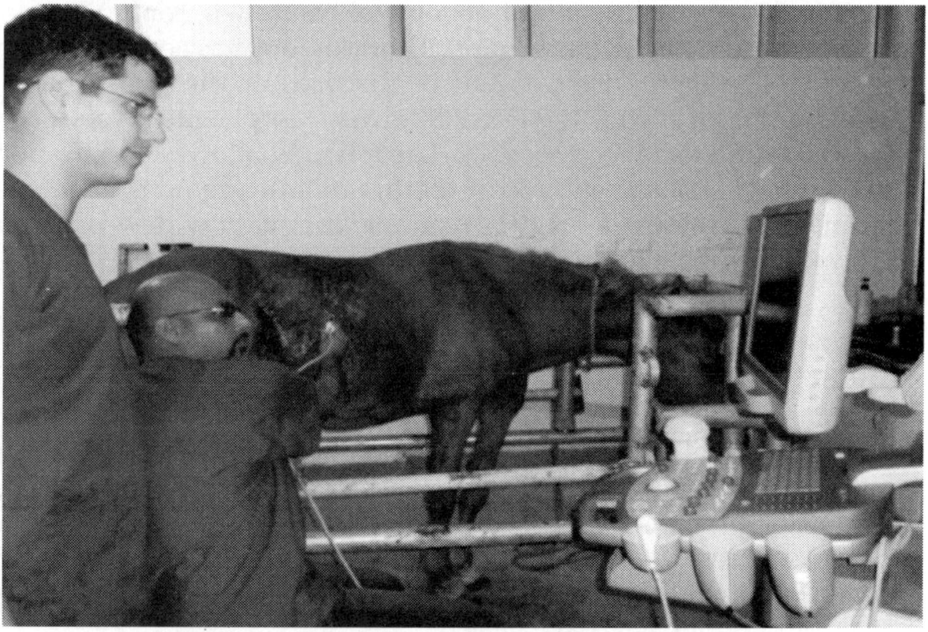

Ultrasonographic abdominal scanning of the horse

Video endoscopy has been used in human medicine for decades, and its use is on the rise in veterinary medicine. Endoscopy is a method of examining the inside of the body using a fiberoptic endoscope. It is an instrument that uses a long, flexible, rubber tube containing fiberoptics that, when combined with a light source, send back to the practitioner a visual picture of the internal structures such as the throat, respiratory tract, gastrointestinal regions, or even joints and the body cavity. Pcopes come in a variety of lengths and sizes. They are typically used for gastrointestinal diagnostics, looking for conditions such as ulcers or hernias. It is also useful for imaging the bladder and intestines. While endoscopes have been commonly used for some time, the addition of video to the technology is relatively new. The video endoscope captures the visuals in a digital form and allows the active video and/or still pictures to be saved and viewed on a computer. This technology is particularly useful in documenting conditions, for education of the client, and consultations.

Laparoscopy has been avaluable diagnostic and therapeutic tool in human clinical medicine. It is now being used extensively in various animal species for research, clinical diagnostic and therapeutic purposes. The most advantageous characteristic of laparoscopy is that it allows direct examination of abdominal cavity with only minimal and superficial surgical intervention. **Thoracoscopy** has been employed for the diagnosis and treatment of diseases of the pleura lung, mediastinum, great vessels, pericardium and oesophagus. **Cystosocpy** is used for urinary tract affections. Laparoscopy allows visualization and biopsy of a large surface of the organ and provides adequate specimen for histopathological diagnosis. It is very widely used for sterilization of small animals.

A veterinarian conducts a bone scan called **Nuclearscintigraphy** by injecting a radioisotope into the bloodstream that is absorbed most fully by areas of increased blood flow, indicating inflammation. Veterinarians can identify areas where soft tissue and bone have suffered damage by noting the areas showing the increased levels of radioactive material. Scintigraphy is also useful in diagnosing bone inflammation where there are no radiographic signs of abnormalities. Dental conditions also can be diagnosed with this modality. In addition, it can differentiate between actively inflamed or painful areas versus old injuries that have healed.

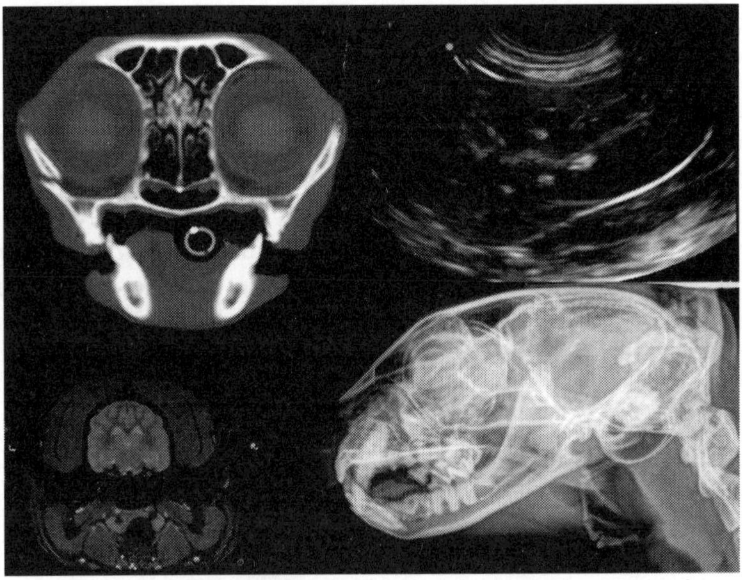

Combination diagnostic imaging

Computer-aided tomography (CT scan, formerly known as CAT scan) is a rotating, focused X-ray beam that is capable of taking "sliced" images of the patient. It does this by using multiple X-ray images to develop a composite image, and it can be used in several areas of the animal's anatomy, including the limbs as well as the head and neck in small animals.

Magnetic resonance imaging (MRI) has only recently become available. It is probably the most expensive of the diagnostic imaging technologies, but it offers many benefits.MRI provides images of the internal body structures using a combination of magnetism, radio waves, and a computer. The image the computer produces is highly detailed and can highlight even small changes of the structures within the body. It is particularly valuable in imaging the brain, spinal cord, joints, stomach, and soft tissues. The modality is painless, allows the patient to avoid the risks of radiation exposure during X-rays, and is an extremely accurate diagnostic tool. It can identify small abnormalities in obscure areas that no other technologies mentioned can image. There are no known risks.

Diagnostic imagings have/had a major impact on the way medicine is practiced in all species. It has made a big difference in the speed and accuracy of diagnosis and treatment. The bar is continually being raised, and who knows what amazing new technology will be available in the near future.

In conclusions, it is emphatically stated that with the fast changing world order, newer tools and technologies with better and better versions in the overall ambit of imaging are being produced. These tools are bound to have greater precisions and faster means for not only quicker and accurate diagnosis but add greater potentials in therapeutics. Therefore diagnostic imaging is crucial for any type of hospital or clinics, independent of location, size and type of resources available.

❑❑❑

Part-III
Abstracted Report, Reference, Publications and Articles having relevance to Veterinary Education

Chapter-14

Abstracts : VCI Sponsored Report on 'Status of Veterinary Colleges in India'-2005

Dr. JITENDRA SINGH BHATIA
Former ADG (EPD) ICAR and Professor of Veterinary on Physiology

It is thought worthwhile to provide certain portions of the report of the study conducted in 2005 that do have relevance in present day context. Some changes at institutional levels diffinately have taken place over the time and thus these may be seen in light of the status as of now.

14.1 Executive Summary

The study examines the inspection as well as the status reports of veterinary colleges in order to identify gaps that exist today with respect to the Minimum Standards of B.V.Sc & A.H. Regulation, 1993. A careful assessment has been made so that institutions become centre of quality training with the capacity and capability of producing professionals who are self confident, self reliant, with knowledge and enriched skills that justifies their relevance and utility to the society. Thus, there is need to take decisive steps in a holistic manner to make corrections in a way that the profession is trying to fulfill its obligation to bring this in line with the changing demand of the society. The profession is not adapting rapidly to the changing needs and is encountering substantial problems on account of shortage of qualified and competent manpower, sub-optimal support system and lacks functional autonomy. Further the governance system is non-conductive to radically step up the needs. The macro-environment with multi channelization in decision-making is too slow in responding and thereby such factors become bottlenecks in overall developmental processes.

An attempt has been made to assess the existing status of veterinary colleges and based on it; some suggestions & recommendations have been made in revitalizing the institution & programs. The proposed recommendations have been made in revitalizing the institution & programs. The proposed recommendation are expected to identify directions for changes needed in veterinary educational programs to equip the professionals to serve the needs of the society in 21th century.

14.1.1 Monitoring and evaluation of academic institutions

Pre -requisite component of a viable institution should have

- Soundness of academic regulation
- Updated syllabus and course curriculum
- Manpower needs - a) Qualified and committed faculty. b) Viable of faculty competence improvement programs.
- Good infrastructure, modern facilities, laboratories instructional farms and associated teaching units.
- Sound financial support, autonomy and good governance system.

The present study has been based upon the aforsand components:

14.1.2 Provision of inspection under VCI regulations

The Council is vested with a power under section 19 of VCI Act 1984 to inspect veterinary institutions and examinations. The council deputes inspectors for the purpose to veterinary colleges and invariably the team visits during the phase of external examinations. **The guideline have been modified and the pro-forma made more comprehensive, however the present system in vogue is mainly targeting towards physical assessment of facilities and procedure adopted in the process of implementation of MSVE rather than objectively evaluating quality of instructions and training being imparted at the institute.** It would me more prudent if instuitions are inspected on certain performance indicators like, quality of graduate output, number of students qualifying at national competitions admissions of foreign students, number of students joining higher education, recognition by acquiring centre of advance studies, national fellows, national professors, resource generation, awards to students, faculty or institutions, faculty getting recognition as visiting scientist, contractual assignments, consultancy services, number and quality of instructional material produced, textbooks published, externally aided projects sanctioned, technologies developed, contributions made for societal built up etc. The emphasis of inspection thus should target for quality assurance and outcome analysis rather than assessing only physical assets. This will add value to inspection and analysis would be more meaningful.

It should also be made mandatory for the institutions to get it externally reviewed of its teaching, research and extension programs through peers. The report of this peer review team and action taken report of the college has to be made available to the VCI.

14.1.3 Curricular Reforms

Course curriculum and academic regulations should have a relevance to the present day needs. Curriculum up-dating is a continuous and dynamic process. It must be ensured that academic programs are revised every five years. The process of revolutionizing the academic curricula is already on and it is expected that there is going to complete transformation of the program that will address to the changing needs of the society.

It is suggested that the course program should have the following three components.

1. Core course (compulsory courses)- 70%
2. Regional specific courses- 20% (Awareness to local/regional issues would be more of a social relevant)
3. Optional courses- 10% (These courses should be specially designed for entrepreneur development skill oriented, business management, social science etc. students should have full freedom to choose courses even across the faculty).

Note : VCI has revised MSVE, regulation 2008. These are in vogue in all veterinary colleges. (Strength and Short falls of 2008 regulations have been dealt in Chapter-2).

14.1.4 Governance

The present education system is highly bureaucratic and is not in tune with the new global environment. There is need to remove all archaic rules and procedures, which are not in tune with the modern times.

Veterinary colleges should be given greater autonomy in terms of academic, financial and administrative management. There should be decentralization of power and empowerment down the line. This will greatly cut short the delay in processing and people become more accountable. There is need to curb the tendency of avoidance or delays in decision making and proper execution. Personnel policies should be re-tuned to attract and retain outstanding teachers/scientists.

14.1.5 Manpower

There is shortage of manpower almost in all colleges. It is more acute in some of the emerging disciplines. The prescribed norms of manpower as per MSVE, Regulations 1993 are high under the prevailing situations and there is a need to revisit VCI regulations on this aspect.

Further the veterinary educational programs have a severe set-back in the present set up since the present policy governing recruitment in SAUs/ICAR is not conducive for attracting talent in R&D programs in this field.

It of course is a healthy trend that veterinary graduates are venturing for self employment and with opening of lucrative avenues in diversified spectrum in public and private sectors, yet **in this transitional phase, if R&D policies are not made attractive, this area is expected to suffer the most.**

There is an emergent need for a policy formulation on manpower planning based upon short term and long term need assessment to man educational institutions.

State Government should immediately create positions on realistic assessment basis and allow the universities/college to go for aggressive recruitment drive.

As a policy initiative, scheme on graduate assistantship, introduction of emeritus (retired) faculty of similar schemes to retain talent, faculty competence improvement programs in emerging disciplines should be formulated.

14.1.6 Reorganization of the institutions

Restructuring of the organization has been proposed from the present departmental concept to divisional concept with a view to drastically cut the cost of establishment, administrative load of the college will be properly shared, decentralization of power would become more meaningful and it will lead to consolidation, prioritization of teaching, research and extension programs and strengthening partnership. These proposed changes, if implemented, would call for amendment to the Act and the Statutes of the universities.(for detail see 14.2.5).

14.1.7 Infrastructure

Present status of laboratories, lecture hall, teaching hospitals, instructional animal farms, and ambulatory services are sub- optimal at most of the colleges. It must be ensured that the institution must have the following basic facilities.

14.1.7.1 Teaching Veterinary Hospital Clinical complex should have access to :

- Outdoor clinic for large and small animals for surgery, medicine and gynecology.
- Operation theaters for surgical and gynecological interventions.
- X-Ray facilities for large with dark room facilities.
- Clinical pathology /diagnostic laboratories.
- Indoor wards/attendant rooms.
- Post mortem complex with animal disposal system and incinerator.
- Availability of major equipments like sono-graphy, endoscope, CCTV, ultra sound, blood gas analyzer, obstetrical equipments laparoscope etc.
- Ambulatory van, animal transport vehicle and carcass disposal trolley etc.

14.1.7.2 Instructional farms

The college must have well developed livestock and poultry instructional units. These units should be independent to that of production farms. It should comprise sizable number of cattle, buffalo, sheep, goat, equine and poultry. In addition depending upon the regional needs, pig, camel, elephant, rabbit etc. should also be made available. The college should also have facility for fodder farm having 25 to 50 acres of irrigated land for fodder production. Animal product technology unit especially for milk and meat evaluation for quality control and processing for products and by-products and there refinement, generation of new technologies for value addition, preservation, packaging and storage for hygienic produce safe for human consumption and feed technology unit especially to demonstrate grinding, pellet making, processing and formulation of animal feed and feed additives and quality control measures etc. should form necessary infrastructure.

14.1.7.3 Building

Many colleges are housed in old buildings, hardly suited to accommodate departments. Remodeling and modernization of the building be accorded priority. Support for construction as well infrastructural development of newly created department may be allocated in phased manner. There is need for construction of girls hostel at veterinary colleges at Bidar, Faizabad, Shirwal, Udgir ,Anand, Raichur, Guwahati etc. Proper examination hall be provided to all veterinary colleges. **(Situations may have been changed as of now).**

14.1.8 Financial support

Through agricultural education that includes veterinary & animal sciences as well, is a State subject and thus it is primary responsibility of the state government to provide basic financial support, yet ICAR which has a role similar to UGC to support and strengthen educational programs and VCI embodied with the responsibility of maintenance of minimum standards of Veterinary education, have to ensure needed support for bringing about improvement in educational standards in the field of veterinary & animal sciences. These two institutions (ICAR & VCI) may participate jointly more often, for overall developments of veterinary education. They may hold structural consultations in assessing the needs in order to build- in support to veterinary colleges at the time of formulation and finalization of plan proposals. **ICAR may also incorporate the suggestions of VCI while allocating and disbursing funds every year. Working these two organizations in tandem is bound to reinforce each other and bring vibrancy to the system in totality for higher efficiency and greater affectivity.**

There is thus a need for an assured multi-dimensional financial support from centre & state governments Mechanisms needs to be worked out for support on continuous basis to enable institutes to implement MSVE, Regulations. In addition, efforts must be directed to generate resources from scientific organization in public and private sectors, industrial houses etc. It must be made mandatory for every institution to generate around 10% of the budget from internal resources through tuition fee, consultancy services, patenting of technologies, sale of produce etc.

State Govt. may also accord operational freedom to the university and colleges to maintain critical manpower level, in each department and in the college.

New colleges may only be created after proper planning manpower needs and making appropriate provisions in the State Plan. State Governments may; in advance apprise VCI of its decision to establish new veterinary college with appropriate financial outlay.

ICAR

ICAR should support liberally "Strengthens & Development grant". Apart from routine grants for conduct of practical, computerization, purchase of text books, preparation of instructional materials, students educational tours etc., and also built in support on continued basis for strengthening veterinary hospitals and diagnostic complex, instructional farm development and purchase operation & maintenance of heavy machinery/plants for milk and meat processing.

One time catch up grant

At present the health of most of the veterinary colleges is not very sound and unless immediate support is provided, the institute may crumble. It is thus very strongly felt that Planning Commission should allocate one time catch up grant to the tune of Rs. 2-5 crores- college during X and XI plans for. **(Need to be calculated as per the prevailing cost index)**

- Up-graduation and modernization of existing facility.
- Creation of new departments including new constructions.
- Faculty competence improvement program in emerging areas of specialization.
- Creation of Centers of Excellence in identified areas.

This support should be over and above the routine grant under the scheme on Development and Strengthening of SAU. **An expert team may be constituted to work out actual requirements.**

State Governments

State Government should ensure for creation of faculty position and immediate recruitment. To supplement the central support of one time catch up grant the state government should provide 25% of the central support for renovation and modernization of buildings. There is also a need for continuous and assured support for contingent expenditure, staff salary and other recurring needs.

VCI

The VCI should continuously strive to maintain liaison with centre and state government, ICAR, scientific organization, universities etc. for garnering desired financial support to veterinary institutions.

SAUs

Universities are required to provide necessary and timely release of funds and granting operational freedom for financial management. Desired autonomy for effective and efficient management of institution is need of the time.

Primary focus: Good institutions, qualified manpower, sound academic programs, modern infrastructure and commensuration financial backup would be purposeful only when our educational system has the capacity to foster a mind set among students. who are analytical, oriented and sensitive to the social and economic issues of the livestock practices in India in the wider context of global developments.

14.2 Suggestions and Recommendations

14.2.1 Creation of manpower-basis problems

State Government has to primarily bear the burden of establishment charges including salary and wages. To get the additional posts created from the state government and then to get approval for filling up the posts is a herculean task. In the present situation of financial crunch, the states are very selective in providing positions. Prior to the lying down of MSVE, regulation, 1993 on an average there used to be 10-12 departments in a college and even in the best of the institution, the posts of professors meant for teaching were not more than 12. In addition, position of associates and assistant professors were roughly about 15 to 20 and 30 to 40 respectively. Additional posts requirements after implementations of MSVE have risen to, 5-7,

10-15, 15-20, respectively for professors, associate professors and assistant professors. This has created a tremendous pressure on the funding agencies. Further these colleges are meeting resistance from within the university, as well as, from the state govt. when it comes to justifying the creation of additional posts on the basis of workload of a teacher. Workload of a teacher is calculated on the basis of UGC guidelines for general universities. Five to seven positions in a department where the total credit load is between 8-12 hrs, seldom meet the yardstick of the government or any other funding agency to create additional posts. The planning process of states usually overlook an integrated responsibility of teaching, research and extension by the faculty of veterinary science. It is thus suggested that manpower needs of the departments may be reassessed based upon credit/contact hour's basis plus additional responsibilities. Further personal promotions schemes through which mass promotions are being carried out in certain universities have tilted the balance in the college/ university. In colloges at Hisar, Punjab and Assam, the base has gone very weak with a heavy top. Large numbers of higher positions especially of professors (through promotion) do not justify creation of additional senior posts and also there is virtual restriction of entry of young talent in the college.

14.2.2 Suggestive Changes in approach

The council may revisit its own recommendations with respect to the staff and may modify these in light of the above but an attempt in this direction requires a careful approach so as to have faculty strength sound enough to carry on the desired responsibilities effectively on long- term basis. Some suggestions in this text are being made after carefully considering all pros and cons.

As a general pattern, it is purposed that, for every three-credit hrs load, there should be one teacher for basic sciences, while for preclinical, para clinical and animal science subjects; it should be 2.5 credits hours per teacher. Additional positions may be provided, if the staff is engaged in clinical/diagnostic or on farm activities. For the faculty engaged in clinical work, one teacher for 2 credits hours be provided. Compensation is made for additional load, as well as time and labor involved in discharging routine duties.

In case of superannuation or for any reason, if it is in knowledge of authorities, the likely creation of vacancy, university may take advance action for recruitment, so that the void likely to be created can be minimized. It of course is required to be assured that the stop gap arrangement (s), if made, has to be regularized by regular appointment while adhering to the prescribed manner of recruitment in a period of 6 months.

14.2.3 Human resource development- Recruitment needs policy formulation

The issue of human resource is complex, firstly availability of manpower in the colleges in low and secondly a recruitment policy to attract talent is not conducive in teaching veterinary institutions and thirdly there is great dearth of qualified and competent manpower in certain emerging discipline like biochemistry, biotechnology, LPT, wild life, laboratory animal management and health; meat hygiene, environmental sciences and information technology etc.

There is need to prepare a national policy on human resource development. It also requires additional financial support extensively for this purpose, in order to fill up the void created in generating competent faculty at veterinary colleges. Some suggestions are put forth in order to cover up the short fall speedily-

1. University may pick up candidates from amongst first five position holders of B.V.Sc & A.H graduate and straightaway induct them on the faculty as teaching assistants/instructors. They will be placed in the department against vacant positions. They should be enrolled for master's degree program in the department. These teaching assistant will partly help in the departments/clinics in conduct of practical and also on part time basis, register for M.V.Sc. In some discipline where faculty to enroll the M.V.Sc is not available in the department/college, they may be deputed to sister colleges to persue education. A memorandum of understanding is required to be developed between institutions for this purpose. Once they attain qualification, they should be screened for the post of assistant professor.
2. There is great need and scope of utilizing the services of retired professional. Presence of experience person would be an asset to young generation. Retired scientist may often be in position to teach economically. The services of retired person should be hired initially for a period of 2 years and they should be paid an

honorarium of Rs. 10-12 thousand/month. These scientists are inducted against vacant positions and in no case number are increased beyond 5 in a college. **(Emoluments of honorarium may be calculated on present cost index).**

N.B. There is going to be no financial burden in implementation of the above proposals since persons engaged in these schemes will be against the vacant posts.

3. College wise contingent plan may also be prepared to depute faculty for training in emerging discipline at a higher centers of learning in India or abroad. Specific budget allocations are required to be made for this purpose.

14.2.4 Entry qualifications of faculty

There is also a need to review the entry qualifications of recruitment in veterinary faculty. Till such time veterinary institutions are able to built up competent veterinarian in emerging discipline, alternate qualification is recommended in order to cover up the immediate gap (wherever it exists) in the following areas.

1. Biochemistry and biotechnology- graduation is biochemistry/ biotechnology with master and doctorate in the subject having specific orientation to animal system.
2. LPM, LPT, animal nutrition, AGB, AH, extension education- graduation is science/agriculture with master/doctorate in the discipline of animal sciences.
3. However in the subject of basic sciences (statistics and computer application, environmental sciences, math, economics and language) basic entry qualification should be graduation is the subject followed by master and doctorate in relevant field.

Alternate qualification would be restricted initially for a period of five years. During this period efforts may be made to trained veterinary graduates to acquire qualifications with a competence to hold the position in the relevant teaching departments. The situation may be reviewed after 5 years.

14.2.5 Creation of departments-Divisional Concept-Proposed

Presently establishment cost in managing departments is very high. Further, with automation the workload of the department office has greatly reduced. It also cannot be denied that there is a heavy load of establishment with the Dean's office in most of the colleges since office support system in the department is very weak. Decentralization of powers to the departmental head is only for a namesake. Thus, in an attempt for right sizing of the institutions and program, should there be a need for bringing changes in organizational setup? As a long term measure, is it feasible to modify the existing structure from the existing departmental concept to divisional concept?

The proposed reorganization has been considered beneficial as

- It drastically cut the establishment cost.
- Decentralization would be meaningful.
- Administrative load would be uniformly divided.
- Integrated approach to teaching the research and extension.

It will help in consolidation, prioritization and strengthening partnership in execution of programs.

Keeping the above in view the following suggestions are put forth.

In a veterinary college there will be five full-fledged Divisions under the administrative control of the Dean.

- Division of basic and social sciences.
- Division of preclinical (biomedical) sciences (foundation courses)
- Division of para-clinical sciences (Supporting Courses)
- Division of clinical sciences.
- Division of production science and product technology.

1. Division of basic and social sciences

The division shall have one main section

- **Veterinary and Animal Husbandry Extension Education**

  In addition it may have the following units (optional)

  - **Bio-statistics, bioinformatics and computer application.**
  - **Live stock economics and marketing.**
  - **Environmental science.**
  - **Any other.**

Head of the division should only be from the discipline of extension education.

N.B. Looking the present status, infrastructure, qualified manpower and requisite facilities in veterinary and AH, extension education is weak, in many of the colleges and thus it is suggested that initially for a period of 5 years the University may also appoint an associate professor as Head of the Division (HOD). However, it should be made compulsory for the University to create a post of Professor and make appointment within 5 years.

2. Division of preclinical (biomedical) sciences (foundation courses)

This division should have two full-fledged sections

- Veterinary Anatomy
- Veterinary Physiology

Those college/universities which have optimum facilities and qualified manpower with a position of Professor in **Veterinary Biochemistry and Biotechnology** may retain it as in independent section while in those colleges where optimum facilities and manpower is yet to be created, it may be made as a sub-section of veterinary physiology but within a span of years, the needed facilities and manpower should be provided. Once it is done, it should be given a status of independent section.

3. Division of para-clinical sciences

This division should have four full-fledged sections

- Veterinary Microbiology
- Veterinary Pathology
- Veterinary Parasitology
- Veterinary Pharamacology

To continue Veterinary Public Health Department as a separate identity is required to be reviewed. The course curriculum of this discipline has three components (milk and meat hygiene and public health, zoonosis and environmental hygiene) APT department also has courses on milk, meat and product technologies. All the courses listed in both the departments are 1+1 credit each. It may be explored to either merge these departments or merged some of the courses to make these as composite courses of 2+1 covering Hygiene, Productions and Product Technology. Likewise Zoonosis course can be merged in veterinary medicine. However, an expert group with subject matter specialists from the concerned disciplines can critically examine and offer suggestions.

4. Division of clinical sciences

This division shall have sections of

- Veterinary Medicine
- Veterinary Surgery and Radiology
- Veterinary Gynecology & Obstetrics

While formulating MSVE, 1993, Regulations, **Preventive medicine** was carved out from Veterinary Medicine and given a status of full-fledged departments. Leaving aside a few colleges, this branch has not attained a status to be retained as an independent unit. **(MSVE, 2008 has again merged these two departments).**

Till such time it acquire a full-fledged unit in terms of infrastructure and manpower it may be made as sub-section of Veterinary Medicine. It must be made mandatory for the university/govt. to provide support to make it as an independent section within a period of 5 years.

It is also suggested that a unit be created in medicine section and appropriates named as veterinary jurisprudence ethics, animal welfare units.

Teaching veterinary clinical complex be treated as an independent section. One of the professors from clinical discipline (Medicine, Surgery and Gynecology) to be appointed as head of Teaching Veterinary Clinical Complex for a fixed tenure. **(It has been made independent department as per MSVE, 2008 regulations).**

5. Division of production science and product technology

This division shall have three sections-

- Live stock Production Management
- Animal Genetics & Breeding
- Animal Nutrition including Feed Technology

Animal Product Technology is made as a subsection of LPM. This subsequently shall have to be raised as an independent section once infrastructure facilities and manpower are provided.

Poultry is one of the fastest growing sectors recording an annual growth rate of more than 10% and is an organized industry. It is contributing 1.2% to the total GDP. Thus there is a need to accord higher priority to this branch of science. **At each college, poultry science may be made a sub-section of LPM department but in a phased manner this should be raised to the status of an independent section.**

Teaching Instructional Farms:- To be managed by LPM department, one of the professors would be assigned the responsibility of managing instructional farm on tenure basis. **(It has been made independent department as per MSUE, 2008 regulation).**

There is a need to spell out working relationship of the sections, within a division. There is a need to retain autonomy of individual discipline on one hand while on the other unification of financial and administrative control for efficient governance is equally important.

14.2.6 Technical support and para professional staff

Support system is invariably very weak at most of the veterinary colleges. Apart from insufficient number of technicians and supporting staff, most of them lack the basic qualifications. Laboratory assistants and technicians in many colleges have been elevated on the basis of time scale promotions and many of them have risen even from clerk and class IV category. X-ray technician, radiographer, stockman, compounder, photographer, curator, computer programmer, operation theatre assistant, audiovisual technician are highly technical positions which are required to be filled from the competent persons.

14.2.7 Laboratories

13.2.7.1 Central instrumentation laboratory: is required to be created at all colleges.

Today such facilities are available only at a few colleges such as Madras, Namakkal, Pantnagar, Hisar and Ludhiana. (Many collages have now created CIF).

There are certain laboratories, which are prerequisite and are needed for different departments but there use is restricted for a limited period. In order to judiciously make use of these laboratories, the possibility of their common use between the departments could be explored. Some suggestions in this context need considerations.

14.2.8.2 Experimental physiology laboratory equipped with kymograph and associated recording system, myograph, respirometer, blood pressure monitor, demonstration table, organ bath, ECG machine etc, is a primary laboratory of veterinary physiology departments, but this laboratory is used for a limited period and that too, in alternate semester. Similar laboratory is needed in veterinary pharmacology. Pharmacology department instead of creating a separate laboratory by duplicating most of the instruments and equipment can share the laboratory of veterinary physiology department.

14.2.8.3 Histopathology, histo-chemistry and tissue processing laboratory can be shared between veterinary anatomy and veterinary pathology. This laboratory can be strengthening by providing CCTV, photo micrographic unit, slides projection aids etc.

14.2.8.3 Analytical laboratory attached to veterinary biochemistry department could be utilized for analytical work needed in physiology, pharmacology, toxicology, medicine etc. Modern gadgets like auto-analyzer, atomic absorption spectrometer, flame photometer etc. could be made available in this laboratory. Likewise **haematology** laboratory can be shared between physiology, biochemistry, pathology and medicine.

14.2.8.3 Apart from these it can be thought of having common facility for :

- Sterilization and autoclaving
- Distillation unit
- Media preparation and culture room
- Computer laboratory with internet facility
- Radioisotopes laboratory etc.

13.2.8.4 There is also a need for museum in the college. It should depict historical events connected with the developments of veterinary and animal sciences, including wild life etc. Technology developments, specimen, handouts, charts, pictures etc. would improve the viability of the college.

14.3 Funding Pattern

Agricultural education, which includes veterinary and animal sciences education as well, is a state subject and therefore major share of funds (between 70-80%) comes from the State Govt. This covers establishment charges, salary and wages contingencies, maintenance of essential services like security, light and water, propulsion charges etc. Occasionally support for construction of building, hostel or purchase of equipment and library strengthening is provided. Major part of the support comes under non-plan while some support is also given under plan scheme.

In addition ICAR provide support primarily under "**strengthening and development grant to SAU's"**. This support to the university is variable between 2-10% of the total grant of the university. This support though is meager, but critical for strengthening educational programs having relevance in preparing graduates with needed skills as well as capacity and capability to meet challenges of the society. The support for ICAR under the aforesaid scheme is provided for contingency for practical, establishment of computer science laboratory, purchase of laboratory equipment, preparation of teaching aids, preparation practical manuals, establishments of central instrumentation laboratory, renovation and modernization of lecture halls with modern teaching technological tools, updating of laboratories and academic blocks. Apart from these, constructions of girls' hostel and renovations of boys' hostel are covered under the scheme. Through other scheme of education division of ICAR viz. national fellow, national professor, emeritus scientist, some of veterinary institutes have taken advantage for infrastructure development, impart trainings and got recognition through its scientist and research output. ICAR has also recognized around 10 departments of veterinary college as *Centers of Advance Studies,* which are serving as a hub to carry out advanced research and imparting trainings to faculty of other institutions. ICAR is also providing support under research (ad-hoc scheme, AICRP and revolving fund) and transfer of technology programs etc. through other subject matter divisions of ICAR. Viable universities/colleges are also getting schemes from other scientific organizations, institutional collaborative projects and to a limited extend from industrial houses and other private sector units. Good universities are generating funds from internal resources to the tune of 5-10% of the total budget.

14.3.1 State Govt. funding

It is a ground reality that no institution is getting sufficient funds to take care of its committed activities. Situation is so grim that certain State Govts. are unable to provide salary to the staff in time. Broadly if analysis is drawn based upon the information provided by the colleges, State grant to veterinary colleges is variable between Rs 2 to 5 crore annually. However, college of Chennai, Hisar and Ludhiana are getting higher allocations while annual grant to Shirwal and Lakhimpur is less than Rs 1 crore. This amount is hardly sufficient to meet the establishment charges and to carry on the essential services including light, water, security, labor, propulsion charges etc. The situation is further compounded by the fact the flow of funds usually from the state Govt. are erratic and untimely. In some of the universities comptroller and finance officers are running from pillar to post in the govt. secretariat, to garner even the committed funds. It, of course, is a fact that, states govt. are under tremendous pressure, due to resource crunch and this is not a temporary setback, but most likely to prevail for long time to come. **There is thus a dire need for financial discipline, public sector institutes need to generate more funds, enters into public private partnerships and programs are to be formulated while eyeing on profitability.** It is an era of consolidation, prioritization and learning to work in partnership. Duplication of efforts has to be curbed, as for as possible and should be target oriented and productive. It, of course, would be erroneous if outputs from educational institutions were weighed only in terms of resource generation. **Building competent human resource is productive investment for future.** In spite of the fact that agriculture sector is contributing 25% of the GDP of which animal husbandry and fish sectors alone are contributing 27% of Agricultural contribution per se which is no way less than any standard. This sector is progressively growing for the last 2 decades at an annual growth rate of about 4.5% compared to 2.2% in agricultural sector. Contrary to it, this sector is getting meager allocation-may it is a central share or state funding or university contributions. It is an established fact that main stay of landless or marginal farmer is animal husbandry. Without undermining the needs for building human resource and infrastructure development in agriculture colleges which are over 70 in numbers in SAU system (and over 100 outside SAU systems), the support to veterinary education is grossly inadequate. **There are only 36 veterinary colleges producing less than 2000 graduates per annum, which are lower**

than the manpower need of the country. Even to these handful of institutions (usually one per state except two in UP, Kerala, Gujarat, Assam, Karnataka, MP, J&K 3 in AP and 5 in Maharashtra) support coming is grossly inadequate. Additional colleges established in Assam, Kerala, UP and Maharashtra is in state of poor health. Apart from these, well-established colleges at Patna, Jharkhand, Mathura, Mhow & Bikaner, which at one time had glories distinctions of being known as ideal educational institutions, are under tremendous pressure for their survival. State Govt. have to be told in no uncertain terms to take immediate contingent measures to bring back these institutions on the road; otherwise time is not far off, when these colleges will crumble of their own. The livestock sector definitely needs a better deal. **(Situation has changed in some colleges over the time).**

14.3.2 ICAR Funding

Educational division of ICAR through its scheme on **"Strengthening and developments of SAU's"** is providing support to State agricultural Universities (SAU'S), Deemed to be universities of ICAR (DU's) and Central universities dealing with Agricultural education (CU's). The support is provided to meet the educational needs, as has already been spelt out. In addition some need based support is provided for construction of girls hostel (100%), renovations and modernization of boys and girls hostel and construction of international hostel (50:50). In addition, to veterinary colleges, specific support on a limited scale has been provided for modernization and updation of of veterinary clinical complex including diagnostic and establishment of animal instructional farms.

During IX plan (rough estimate) veterinary colleges by and large got support between Rs 1-2 crores which forms 20-30% of the total grant allocated to university. Although support coming from **"Strengthening and development" grant is meager, but it remained critical. This support has been very handy in revamping education though at a limited scale so far and thus there is need to scale up this grant proportionate to its growing requirements. There is also a necessity to cover up some specific activities pertinent to veterinary colleges. These readjustments do not call for structural changes in the scheme but are possible in the overall ambit of the scheme in vogue.**

Keeping the aforesaid activities in view, average support under development grant to veterinary education in a plan period would

be around Rs. 200-250 crores which can be conveniently accommodated within the approval of X plan outlay.

Apart from the one time catch up grant between 2.5- 5.0 crores be given to each veterinary college in this and next plan periods to cover up severe shortfall in infrastructure, renovation of old buildings, animal farms, construction of additional blocks to accommodate new disciplines etc. Special provision to be given of 100 crore during the remaining period of this plan is made available for this purpose and this should be continued at least in XI plan.

14.3.3 Strategic approaches for growth of veterinary institutions

Some suggestions

Though veterinary education is a state subject and institutions are created and primarily supported through state funds but sustenance of the programmes, attaining uniformity of academic standards and remedying regional imbalances are national concerns. There are wide variations between number of institutions, manpower availability, infrastructural requirements and commitments in terms of maintenance of minimum standards of education being imparted in veterinary sciences. Though there are few colleges, which have the capacity and capability to award high quality education, and meeting international standards but equal number of institutions are there, which do not have any of the basic prerequisite facilities and are not worth considering these as a viable component of system. Thus, veterinary education, if viewed in totality in the country, it gives a very dismissal picture. In order to tone up the system and to streamline educational institutions, retuning policies and programme, to make it user friendly and enhancing social relevance to it, united efforts required. A few steps in the connection are suggested, however, council may develop its own course of action, as it deem proper, in this context.

14.3.3.1 VCI may circulate status document after updating it with other vital transformation it has brought over the time, to all agencies of centre and state govt. connected with AH development programs and impress upon them to share the concern of VCI so that desirable dimension to the educational programs are added at a faster pace.

14.3.3.2 Council may appraise the status of veterinary educational institutes to the Union Minister of Agriculture and impress upon it to intervene. Agriculture minister may convene a meeting of State Animal Husbandry Ministers, Secretaries of AH departments of GOI and State

Govts, Vice Chancellor of SAU's and other stakeholders. VCI may make detailed presentation in this meeting. This body after in depth analysis may take implements able decisions. The agenda for the meeting should address to :

i) The developing mechanisms of support on continuous basis to the colleges to enable them to implement VCI regulations effectively.

ii) New colleges may only be created after planning proper manpower needs and making appropriate provisions in the state Plan for an ideal institution. State Govts may in advance apprise VCI of its decision to establish veterinary college and commitment made for the new college including financial outlay.

iii) State Govt. may also accord operational freedom to the university to maintain critical manpower level, in each department and in the college.

14.3.3.3 Since VCI is embodied with the responsibility of laying down the MSVE and ICAR has the mandate to provide critical financial support to fulfill its obligations to impart quality educations, these two institutions may participate jointly more often, in overall developments. They may hold structural consultations in assessing the needs in order to build in support to veterinary colleges at the time of formulation and finalization of Plan proposals. **ICAR may also incorporate the suggestions of VCI while allocating and disbursing funds every year. Working these two organization in tandem is bound to reinforce each other and bring vibrancy to the system in totality for higher efficiency and greater effectively.**

14.3.3.4 Vice Chancellor's conference organized annually by education division of ICAR provides a platform to discuss issues pertaining to educational reforms in agricultural universities and significant decisions are taken which facilitate easy implementation throughout the country. President and Secretary VCI should be invited in the meeting. **In the next meeting of Vc's, while giving priority to this branch of science, one session may be earmarked to discuss veterinary education.** Dean's of the colleges should also be invited for the session.

14.3.3.5 The Chancellors of SAU's may also be appraised of the ground realities of veterinary education in his state *vis a vis* the national scenario. He can, on one side, ensure through the Govt. to garner needed support, while on the other impress upon the universities to initiate all effective steps to implement MSVE, regulation, 1993, in letter and spirit. Amendments to the university status, rule, regulation or ordinances if some provisions are coming in the way of implementation of VCI regulations, may be brought about speedily.

14.3.3.6 Presently in most of the universities, Dean, HOD other academic management positions are rotational and thus there is need to develop mechanisms to orient as well as sensitize them at regular interval on various facets of managing veterinary institutions. ICAR is also structuring similar meetings for academic manager in SAU's. In case, such events are conducted as a joint venture, ICAR can built- in complete financial support for organizing meets through development grant. Such approach would be meaningful and collective approach would ignite a spark to the entire machinery involved in the process of strengthening and revamping veterinary education.

Concluding Statement

14.5 - Veterinary Council of India is a statutory authority to lay and maintain the minimum standards of veterinary education, but more than this, it has its obligations to ensure that veterinary institutions are fully equipped to effectively discharge their responsibilities. It, of course, cannot be denied that onus of implementation of statutory regulations/ provisions remains with organizations adopting these, yet VCI, being the central pivotal force, if it extend strength and support; it would be catalytic for rejuvenating institutions. For achieving it, a continuous dialogue with centre and state govt. funding agencies and universities is time demanding. The Council should move forward a national perspective or strategy of veterinary education in order to make veterinary institutions capable of producing human resource that has potentials to fulfill aspirations of present day need as well as capacity and capability to adjust to ever changing needs of the society. The profession is encountering multi-dimensional challenges. These challenges provide opportunities for the profession to improve the quality, effectiveness and usefulness of its services to the society.

14. B Additional Documents / Reports having Relevance to the Veterinary Education

I. Veterinary Council of India (VCI)

1. IVC Act, 1984 (52 to 1984)
2. VCI - Minimum Standards of Veterinary Education – (B.V.Sc & AH) Regulations, 1993
3. VCI (1995) - Human Resource Development in Veterinary Profession
4. VCI - Minimum Standards of Veterinary Education – (B.V.Sc & AH) Regulations, 2008
5. VCI - National Seminar on "Veterinary Education and Practice - Present Status and Future needs to Meet the Emerging Challenges" 21-22 September, 2007, Bangalore
6. VCI - National Seminar on "Strategies of Strengthening Veterinary education and Practice sector's December, 2008, Hyderabad

II. Animal Husbandry Department, GOI

7. Census Report (2007 & 2012)
8. Annual Report (2013-14) of Department of Animal Husbandry, Dairying and Fisheries, Ministry of Agriculture, GOI
9. Report of the Expert Committee of Veterinary Education of Department of Animal Husbandry, Dairying and Fishers, Ministry of Agriculture, GOI (2014).

III. Indian Council of Agricultural Research (ICAR)

10. Dr. M.S. Swaminathan Committee report on 'Education for Agriculture-Bridge to a Century of Hope on the Farm Front' (1997).
11. Policy for Higher Agriculture Education in India 2013. Agriculture Education Division ICAR, New Delhi
12. Veterinary Education in India by Dr.P.N. Bhat In 50 years of Agriculture Education in India ICAR Editor S.L. Mehta and B.S. Mathur (2000).
13. ICAR Model Act for Agricultural Universities of India (2009)
14. Dean's committees of ICAR (1972, 1984, 1994, 2005)

IV. National Academy of Veterinary Sciences (NAVS)

15. Proceeding of NAVS Workshop on Veterinary Education for Human Resource needs in Animal Husbandry Sector Jaipur, Rajasthan, (2013) Jointly organized by The Rajasthan University of Veterinary and Animal Science, Bikaner and National Academy of Veterinary Sciences (India), New Delhi.

16. NAVS Policy Paper II. 'Human Resource needs for Veterinary and Animal Sciences' (in press).

V. National Academy of Agricultural Sciences (NAAS)

17. Models of Public Private Partnership In Agricultural Bio-Technology: Brain Storming -NAAS (2007)

18. A Road Map to Transform Agricultural Education to Reshape India's Future: National Academy of Agricultural Sciences, NASC New Delhi, 2014. NAAS edited by R.B.Singh.

VI. OIE and other documents

19. (a) Resolutions adopted at 2nd Global Conference on Veterinary Education Lyon, France 13-14 May 2011

(b) Report on the meeting of OIE, AD-Hoc group on VETERINARY EDUCATION, Paris11-13 January, 2012.

(c) Guide lines for Veterinary Statutory body TWINNING Projects, August 2013 and September 2013.

(d) Veterinary Education Core Curriculum, OIE guidelines September, 2013.

VII. Others

20. The Foresight Report: Envisioning the Future of Veterinary Medical Education. Journal of Veterinary Medical Education-Special Issue Volume 34(1), 2007

21. FICCI Report "Accelerating Public Private Partnership in India-Submit 2012

22. Human Resource Development Strategies on for Veterinary Profession-An outlook by Janardhan Challa, NAARM, Hydrabad

23. India, Human Resource development relevant to Veterinary Service Requirement. II. Continuing Veterinary Education in India: Challenge ahead by Prof. (Dr. Rama Kumar,V & Ajit Maru

14.C Publications of the Author

1. Bhatia, J.S (1997) A Scenario of Veterinary Education in India. Short course on Veterinary Educational Technology, CCS HAU, HISAR
2. Bhatia, J.S (1997) Veterinary Education in India- A perspective. Short course on Veterinary Educational Technology, CCS HAU, HISAR
3. Bhatia, J.S. (2011). Veterinary education in India-a critique: NAAS News Letter 2011, July-September, page 3-6.
4. Bhatia, J.S. (2012). Major issues concerning Veterinary Education in India: University Today. New Delhi, May 2012.
5. Bhatia, J.S. (2013 a) Future Technical Human Resource requirements of Livestock Sector. NAVSI Convention LLRVAS, HISAR (jan28-29, 2014)
6. Bhatia, J.S. (2013 b) Human Resource Development -A Challenge in Veterinary Sector-Personal communication.
7. Bhatia, J.S. (2013 c) Human resource a key component for growth- Personal Communication.
8. Bhatia, J.S. (2013 d). Time demands re-tuning of Veterinary Education: Paper presented in National Symposium of SAPI, Mathura, Nov, 2013.
9. Bhatia, J.S.(2013e) Clouds on Veterinary Education-(Critical time to cement wedges)
10. Bhatia, J.S. (2014). Some suggestions on Standard Operative Procedures (SOP) for inspection of Veterinary Institutions and Colleges as per provisions of the IVC Act, 1984.
11. Yadav, M.P and Bhatia, J.S (2014) Transforming Veterinary and Animal Sciences Education for Reshaping India's economy In 11th Agricultural Science congress Transforming Agricultural education for Reshaping India's future.

❑❑❑

Prof. (Dr) Jitendra Singh Bhatia,

BVSc&AH, MSc (AIIMS) PhD,
FNAAS, FNAVS (I)

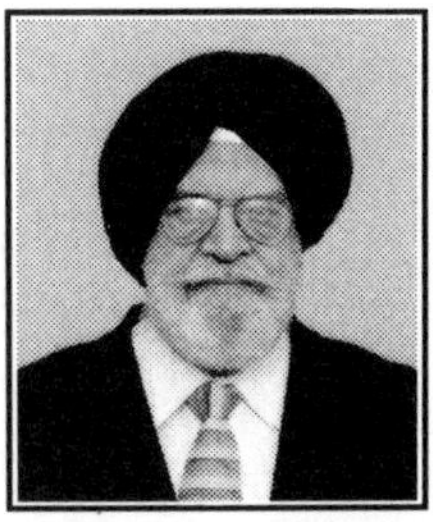

Born in SIMLA on 29.05.1942

Qualification: Educated at College of Veterinary and Animal Science, BIKANER 334001,BVSc&AH 1965, AIIMS, M. Sc (1974), Sukhadia University, Udaipur, Ph.D(1984)

Professional experience: Former ADG (education development & planning) ICAR, Controller of Examinations with Rajasthan Agricultural University, Bikaner, Professor of Veterinary Physiology, CCS HAU Hisar, Apollo College of Veterinary Medicine, Jaipur and presently working at Khalsa College of Veterinary & Animal Sciences, Ram Tirth Road, Amritsar-143 002

Professional contributions: Professional experience of 50 years of working as faculty member, academic manager and policy planning and plan formulations at Center and State Governments. Remained actively involved in teaching at UG and PG level and guided students at master's and doctorate level.

Associated with highest managemental and academic bodies with agricultural/ veterinary universities till date.

Member of various national committees: Peers Review committees (PRC) of the Universities, Scientific organizations,. Accreditation committees, Quinquennial review committee (QRT), selection boards, search committees and members of the scientific & professional councils and fellows of National societies.

Major area of research: Rumen Physiology with special reference to Camel ecology, Neuro-endocrinology with particular reference to alterations of hypothalamic mechanisms in diabetics. Handled externally funded scientific projects as Principal Investigator and Co-Investigator

Assignments at hand: Member of Board of Management of a Veterinary (RAJUVAS) and an Agricultural University (CSK HPKVV), member of Peers review committee of the Maharashtra Animal and Fishery Sciences University (MAFSU), Nagpur. Professor and Head, Department of Veterinary Physiology & Bio-Chemistry, and Academic Coordinator, Khalsa College of Veterinary and Animal Sciences, (KCVAS) Amritsar.

Publications: Besides, 50 scientific publications in National and International Journals of repute, published and circulated more than 25 articles on Veterinary Education and is regularly contributing articles of professional interest in News Letters, Journals, Magazines, Periodicals and have presented lead papers, key note address at National and International conferences.

E-Mail bhatiajs05@rediffmail.com and bhatiajs05@gmail.com

Communication address Q No.8 Khalsa College campus, Near Heritage Guest House, GT Road, Amritsar, 143001

Delhi address B-101, Mandakini Apartment, Plot-3-C, Sector-2, DWARKA, New Delhi-110 075. Mobile 91-9316612588